SKINNY

WOMEN

ARE NOT

CREATED

EQUAL!

Weight Loss Surgery in a

Commercial Diet World!

DR. TERRI A. SIMMONS

DEDICATION

I dedicate this book to all of the woman who are
striving to be their best selves.

Skinny Women Are Not Created Equal

By Dr. Terri A. Simmons

ISBN-9781793120076

Published by Carriage House
and Dr. Terri A. Simmons

www.carriagehousepublisher.com

drterrisimmons@gmail.com

PRINTED IN THE U.S.A.

TABLE OF CONTENTS

PREFACE

Many people who have known me for most of my life, who see me now, have said to me, "What happened to youuu?!!" When I tell them that I lost more than 120lbs. they say, "Girl, that's wonderful! How'd you do it?" When I say, "I decided to have weight loss surgery..." They back up, "Wwwwhat? Really? You took the easy way out!" Surgery is never the easy way out. After the surgery you have a lifetime of work to keep you at the weight that you desire. If you decide to take on a commercial diet program, you still have to follow a plan to make it work.

So to say that surgery is the easier road, is absolutely ridiculous! The only difference, in my opinion is that you were desperate and serious enough to allow doctors to go into your body and alter your stomach so that you are forced to begin the change that you desire. If you don't comply, it's painful both physical as well as mental, but I'll go into that in later chapters.

The purpose for this point-by-point, step-by-step book is to encourage and inspire you to discover who you are. I don't want you to look at the big picture and get overwhelmed, just look at the little picture and work on that a moment at a time.
While there are many stories out there, I want you to learn from my experiences and hopefully something in my story will help you to conquer your weight concerns once and for all.
I HAVE REALLY BEEN WHERE YOU ARE.

Maybe you have already had weight loss surgery and it was successful. But maybe you've had it and you've gained your weight back. Perhaps you are not going that route at all and have decided to try one of the many commercial diet programs out there. Or maybe you have tried them all, like me, and nothing worked and you are at a loss.

Maybe you are considering weight loss surgery but the thought frightens you. Whatever the case, my endeavors are to give insight and information on my journey through commercial diets and then through surgery and you make the decision on your own.

**For nearly 40 years I have absolutely been that "Fat Girl".
I know what I'm talking about!**

So please, sit back, get comfortable and enjoy. Oh, one last thing... you will find that I have highlighted and/or underlined various statements because I want you to really, really remember them! I'd like you to get out your own highlighter and pen and do your own underlining and highlighting too...and please write your notes in the margin!!   ***

INTRODUCTION

I lived with weight issues for more than 35 years of my life. I went on every diet program known to man. I even had **Two Life Memberships to "Jenny Craig...TWO"** and neither one of them worked! I joined Woman's Workout World, Bally's, LA Fitness and bought all of the Billy Blanks, Extreme Work Out and so many promising Dance, Yoga, and _"BURN THAT FAT NOW"_ tapes but all they did was cash my checks! I needed real help from real people who had really been where I was and not only that, I needed a **serious mind change** which none of them addressed! I didn't need a 110lb counselor who had never experienced her thighs rubbing together nor a counselor who had never worn a girdle! I didn't need a fitness trainer telling me, "That's the reason you're fat, now 10 more!"

I had high blood pressure, diabetes, and panic attacks all the time. I was tired of walking, tired of standing, tired of sitting and tired of sleeping. I wore a 44FF Bra, which was hard to find unless I looked in the construction section of major department stores or in mail order magazines, and then you are talking real money and constant returns because they just didn't fit! I was just tired....and miserable all the time!

My turning point came when I got on a plane to attend a business meeting and the seatbelt didn't fit. The woman in front of me asked the stewardess for a seatbelt extension but I refused to ask for one. I folded my gut up, sucked it all in and flew 5 hours absolutely disgusted with myself for the last time!

10 years later I had weight loss surgery which was a marvelous beginning but **WAS NOT AN END!!!** It worked perfectly for 6 or 7 years and took me from a

near 300lb squishy-mommy, well I was actually a 270lb, size 28W mammoth- mommy to a 125lb, size 4 petite itty-bitty babe!

Then life hit and hit hard and I began putting the weight back on and thought, "This wasn't supposed to happen!" This happened because although the doctors changed my insides, **I didn't change in my thinking about food!** And when you don't have that mind change, you will go back to your old habits and your body remembers and will return to its former state.

I owned a thriving 24 hr. Group Home and Day Care business for 30 years, I was also a Professor for Chicago City Colleges for 15 years, as well as a national author and publisher.

I was stressed because I was hustling and working hard. I was making a lot of money, 6 figures a year but, I was getting paid from 100% for my own efforts. I had not yet learned how to get myself positioned to get paid from 1% of 100 people's efforts, and neither did I know anything about having a Plan "B" so that as I got older I wouldn't have to work so darn hard. I was stressed and worked and worked and ate and struggled and ate and worked myself up to nearly 300lbs of bad health, depression and frustration.

I had just entered the world of Multi-Level Marketing which was fast becoming my business of choice and promising to supersede all of my other incomes. I wanted to get off the roller coaster and this new business would pave the way for that Plan "B" stuff that I just spoke about, however I had amassed so much weight and so many health issues that I couldn't even work the new business effectively.

SKINNY WOMEN ARE NOT CREATED EQUAL

Not only did I have high blood pressure, diabetes, panic attacks, I had numbness in my feet and fingers. I had blotchy skin, my thighs rubbed until they burned all the time and I lived with knee pain and indentations in my shoulders from my bra. I had sleep apnea and a real bad body image.

What made things worse was all the money I was making, from the businesses I already had and now the new business that I had begun, I was still broke! That's why I was depressed and frustrated. I was working and working and trying to live the American dream and getting fatter and fatter doing it! But I wouldn't dare let anybody know it. I was living a lie and proud to be pulling it off!! Stupid!

Along with all of the crazy things I have tried, I'm embarrassed to say that I was so desperate that I went to what was known as the "Fat Doctor" of the South Side and got a series of pills that gave me too much potassium, dehydrated me, took away my appetite and sped up my metabolism all at the same time. I felt like a nervous, numb cartoon character, you know, the one who runs into a tree and falls out and then sees stars and goes, "yadda-yadda-yadda?" I was like that all day, every day for months. I couldn't continue to live like that either!!

I even remember getting a prescription for pills from my primary doctor that blocked fat from the foods that I ate. But the oil had to escape somewhere... and when I got up from sitting anywhere...there the oil was! I actually considered keeping up with this prescription and wearing adult diapers to keep my clothes clean and keep me from embarrassment. I was so desperate! Desperately nuts!! There had to be a change! I was not living! I was in a silent misery. Susan Powder said, "Stop the madness!

To prepare me for life after surgery, I had great nutritional education for 6 months prior to surgery, but I didn't hold onto it. Not only that, but there had to be an understanding of my particular needs. What I need now, TODAY is not what I needed 10 years ago. Neither do I have the same "cookie cutter needs of John B or Betty Q like what they dish out at the popular weight loss centers. Everything is the same for everybody who comes through their doors or lands on their website. That's one of the major mistakes of these fad diets. Every single body is different and should be treated as such by a personal counselor or that EDUCATED person who had BEEN THERE and promises to take the client from point "A" all the way through to point "Z".

I'm "39.95" (that means I didn't want to be 40), and have been 39.95 for 16 years, (that means I'm now 56), but my body is different now and requires different things.

So the pounds came back on and one day I looked up and I was JUST UNDER 200lbs! Being disgusted was mild! Nevertheless, I was introduced to a concept called feeding your blood type and a whole new way of eating which includes being on top of all vitamins and supplements. When you are a bariatric patient you don't absorb all of the necessary nutrition, therefore you must take your vitamins and supplements to remain healthy. You are absolutely fooling yourself if you think you don't need them, but I'll talk about that later as well.

My mission now is to reach as many individuals, especially women who have struggled and who are struggling with their weight issues. I want to talk with you if you have had surgery and have begun to gain that weight back, or if you are thinking about surgery because you don't know what else to do. Don't go out and purchase or sign up for another diet anything because ***diets do not work!!***

Based on my knowledge and my experiences and because I can't walk with everybody who desires my help, I created this book because I want to walk with you through your process of reinventing yourself. No matter how many times you've tried to lose weight in the past, you have the right to do it again. It's just a matter of how, when and what is the best method for you! ***

44-FF IS NOT A HAT

My girlfriend, Gayle of almost 30 years wanted to return the favor and buy me a beautiful, lacy bra and panty set like I had purchased for her as a gift for Christmas. Hers was easy, she wore 34A, so the "children's section" was loaded with cute stuff...lol!

She set out to buy me what she thought would be really cute and lift my spirits. I had only ever worn expensive, white construction bras since my breasts had always been so very large and big, box, white, granny panties were my choice.....Hey, don't judge me!

I mean, back then my thought was what's the point in wearing anything else other than white panties if I can't get cute bras to go with them? She felt sorry for me so she really wanted me to feel good about myself and wanted to surprise me.

Without my help or input, she and her daughter, Maria went to one of those "Passion" stores to find a passionate set of matching under garments for me. She explained to me her adventure into "Hat-land!" She said, "There it was, hanging on the rack, in living color, Pumpkin Orange and had black inset

lace...Beautiful!" But she had no idea what size I wore.
The biggest size they had hanging there on the rack
was a 44-FF. She said to her daughter, "Surely, Terri
doesn't wear this size, it's so big!" And before she
knew it, she had placed it on her head as a hat and
paraded herself over to the mirror to admire how
lovely the lace graced her brow!

My cup size was definitely large enough to be a hat,
that was where I was at the time, but she didn't know
it. I remember feeling terribly embarrassed and
thankful at the same time. However, I know now that
there is nothing to be ashamed of. My grandmother
was a 54-G so it's in my genes to have "Big Girls!"
When I lost the weight, I lost the hat and the big girls!
Today I am a proud 34D with no surgery. Actually,
they aren't really big girls any more, rather "Old
Women!"

Years after my weight loss Gayle and I and about 55
or 60 other women went to be part of a talk show
audience in the city. We had to ride the bus that was
provided by our host who was also treating all of us to
lunch and there was a tremendous wait ahead of us.
So she and I and the other women sat and waited and
made the best of our time on the bus. We all began to
chat with each other and talk about all sorts of things.

Well....Gayle and I began talking about underwear and
as I began to show her and explain about the straps
on my bra, I looked down and since I had lost so
much weight, my "Old Women" were puddling inside
my bra! With so much skin left over from the 44-FF, I
would just pour them into my smaller 34D! I said, "Oh
look, see this is what I was trying to explain to you on
the phone, my puddles!" She kind of leaned in and
looked into my shirt and saw my puddles and we both
broke into hysterical laughter. The ladies in front of us
and the ladies behind us kind of stopped their

conversations to ask us what we were laughing so hard about which made us laugh harder.

I began to explain the puddling and they began to laugh. Soon half of the bus was laughing over my puddles. Why? They could understand and some could relate. It was funny, I was free to tell such a story and certainly there were other stories springing from that one and for that short time on the bus, I was everybody's friend.

And while I'm at it, I'll tell you this story too... I had a friend to come over to fit me for the right size bra. She owned a Corset Shop and wanted to really give me a good fitting bra. So she came in with this suite case filled with all sizes of white braziers rolled up in their individual sleeves. They were labeled and before I could go to "Z", I randomly yanked up "60-Q". Holy Moses!! That was enough for me. I didn't want to see "Z" anything!

It's nothing now to run into a little store and pick up a bra and panties if I'm out of town and forget to pack underwear because I'm in a hurry...hey it happens! Back then, I had to pay tall dollars for heavy duty braziers, but today, it's nothing at all. It still makes me go, "WOW!" That's something that skinny women take for granted. A $10 bra would disintegrate under my arms in a matter of hours when I was at my heaviest weight. Today, $10 bras are part of my wardrobe! ***

<u>SUCK IT UP</u>

I was getting on a plane heading out on a business trip from Chicago to Atlanta. The woman seated in front on me was very overweight and didn't even bother to try to put the seatbelt across herself so as the stewardess walked pass, she asked the woman if she wanted the seatbelt extension....(What? seatbelt extension?!? I had never heard of such!!) The woman was comfortable with the questions and said, "Oh yes please. Thank you."

In the meantime, I was thankfully sitting in the window seat and hiding as I was forcing the seatbelt to fit across my belly. It absolutely would not fit. I was not going to ask that stewardess for that doggone extension. I'd rather ride the 2 hours in complete agony and discomfort than to admit I could not fit within those 24 inches.

It was then I made the decision to change my life. Wearing size 28w clothing is embarrassing when you live inside a 5ft. 2in. frame and waddle everywhere you go and **YOU KNOW YOU WADDLE!**

I was out of breath and plum tired all the time. I had scars from my bra burning into my skin. I was tired of sitting in the back seat of anyone's car and the seatbelt not fitting. I would fake it and tuck the buckle under my stomach as if it were securely fastened. When I got back home I'd eat from frustration and wasn't even aware of it.

Obsessive eating becomes a disorder and if your genes are susceptible to it, obesity becomes your disease. This way of eating happens very early. It begins with candy, chips or even fruit as a kid. It's not necessarily what you're eating but *why* you're eating. It's the eating that becomes the habit. Later you replace the fruit for the jelly donuts.

An obese person lives in embarrassment and doesn't even know it, maybe they don't realize it. Often other people observing their awkwardness or uncomfortableness and are embarrassed for them. They don't want to admit it but getting on a bus and hitting the other passengers in the head with their hips and their bag as they pass by is not only irritating to the fellow passengers but if they have a conscience it is embarrassing to the one who is obese. And Lord, when they finally do sit down, they are sweating and huffing and puffing something awful.

I remember finally sitting down after wrestling my way into the waiting room and through a crowd of mothers and babies in a doctor's office with my four little boys, three walking, and one in a car seat. I came in virtually disturbing every atom in the atmosphere! Car seat, diaper bag, children, plastic toys, crying, running noses, bottle and pacifier and making so much noise! I was panting so bad the mother sitting next to me thought I was going to have a heart attack! I was sweating hard, breathing hard, holding myself up with my arm on the back of the other chair and had no breath to tell my boys to sit down. My oldest, Mike-Mike who was perhaps 7 years old at the time, looked at me and saw that I was in distress and corralled his two younger brothers together at my knee as best he could until I could come back to life!

We all have seen overweight people just wrestle with themselves to get from one place to another in a room. Even though I had kids with me, we have seen big people go through this without any children and we have felt embarrassed for them or sometimes annoyed by them.

If you have not lived in that place, you could not possible understand. But if you have lived in that "fat sack" for any length of time, you don't realize that you are offending or worrying people and disturbing the atmosphere by invading their space. You are just trying to do what you do and live like everybody else. Certainly it's not an obese person's intention to offend another person with their presence, however it's rather difficult when the world is not set up to always accommodate the larger population. The movie theater, that airplane seats, the dentist office, and so on... some of them are doing more to accommodate larger people, but there still are so many uncomfortable situations where overweight people get in the way of others. I don't mean to say it that way, and even though it may not be your fault that you are obese, it is still an invasion on the other person's space.

There is no thought to where the skinny girl will sit on a plane, in a crowded room, on a bus or will she fit down through the movie seats or in a small car? She just bounces on through and takes a seat. She has no thought that she is invading anyone's space. From the seats in the movie theater to the sanitary pads, the world is fitted for the size 10 woman. Certainly, as I said, some things are moving to accommodate a larger person because of the world's changing needs but most of the world still caters to right handed and a size 8-10, nude colored woman! ***

EVERYBODY'S FRIEND

I wanted to lose weight so desperately that I found the money to sign up with every program out there. Back in 1985 when my oldest son was a baby and I went from 110lbs to 229 AFTER delivery. I was desperate and paid for a "Lifetime" Membership to Jenny Craig Weight Loss Center near my job in the City.

They promised they would help me shed those 119 seriously unwanted pounds. My counselor's name was Mickey and she reassured me that she was the most successful Weight Loss Counselor at the Center there and she would be coaching me all the way! Not even 3 months later that Center closed and Mickey was nowhere to be found!

So I moved onto another Center closer to home. The counselor there said, "Yep, I am the most successful Weight Loss Counselor here and have been for the last 14 years! I will be with you every step of the way!" This was a bit eerie. She was nearly saying the same thing Mickey said. Hmmmm.... are they trained to say this? To make matters worse, this counselor could not have ever been 100lbs *even if she were wet and pregnant!* So how could she sympathize or empathize with me? How could she have ever felt what I was currently feeling? She was very pretty and well put together but I'm stretching it to guess that she was even 85lbs!

Anyway, I told them that I was a lifetime member from another Center and they took me right on in. I purchased the food for the week....$200 worth and still had to buy the extra stuff and food for my baby and husband. After a few weeks, it just didn't seem smart. Nonetheless I stuck it out. I walked on a track every day, ate the "almost" tasty Jenny foods and paid close attention to my intake.

After 6 months I barely lost 25lbs. which was a grave letdown to me at the time. So I gave it up and instead I had another baby....and gained 69lbs.! So let's see, I was 110lbs. at the start, I gained 119lbs. which put me at 229lbs. post baby. Then I lost 25lbs. which put me at 204lbs. but I then gained 69lbs. that landed me at 273lbs. Holy Smokes!

When you are big, you tend to be jovial and funny and everybody's friend. I wanted to be liked by everybody because I didn't like myself. In a crowd of people I didn't have an opinion because I didn't want to go against the grain of others. In private I cried and cried a lot. I remember asking God to help me figure out how to lose weight. When I thought he didn't answer fast enough, I had another baby! Don't get me wrong, I love my children. All 5 of them are grown and beautiful now. As a young mother struggling with my weight back then, having babies was what I was good at, and I found my comfort and affirmation in my children and my husband. The world is cruel and if you are not careful and emotionally tough the world will show you just how much you DO NOT measure up to the set standards of beauty.

That's why, at the printing of this book, it is estimated that an individual personally spends nearly $16,000 a year on some kind of weight loss program in the U.S. and as a whole, nearly $70,000,000 is spent on it. Every one of them are trying to fit into that model of what beautiful, healthy, handsome, glamorous, gorgeous and "sho-nuff fine is! Even the skinny chicks are trying to keep up with the skinnier and more beautiful babes. The wafer thin and boney ones are not thin or boney enough and the tanned and dark ones are not toasted enough. If you let the magazines and commercials dictate to you what beauty should be, you will never, ever get there!

Avon Beauty Products were my weakness. I never could get enough of the lipsticks. When I saw the models on the pages wearing the new shade of Rosier Reds or Pinkier Pinks I just had to have it. But for what? To have my lips look like theirs? Over a short period of time I had accumulated hundreds of shades only to throw them away and start over. What a waste of money. The last thing I want to say about that is....advertising really worked on me!!!

There comes a point where you are tired of being everybody's friend on a fake level. All you really want is one or 2 real friends who feel you and who know where you are emotionally. Who may or may not be where you are physically but who also want to go where you want to go, support you and don't want to hinder you. In fact, they want destiny just as badly for you as they want it for themselves.

It may be like finding a needle in a haystack but there is someone out there looking for you just like you are looking for them, if you are really looking for them. Fake friends are like credit cards, they seem to be easy to get, charge you a lot of interest and are a headache in the end! ***

FAT FRIEND-SKINNY FRIEND

I had 2 best friends as a young adult. Geraldine was extremely overweight and Hanna was paper thin. Whenever I was out with Gerry, she wanted to eat all the time. One day we were on our way out for dinner. On the way, she stopped into the local drugstore to pick up a box of granola bars and a liter of diet cola. As we drove to the restaurant, she proceeded to open and eat all 8 bars and down the cola. In the middle of her feast, she did offer me some, but I declined. I did ask her why she was eating since we were on our way to dinner. Her reply was that this was just to keep the hunger away and get her to dinner. It wasn't much and won't spoil her appetite! At dinner, she had a Porterhouse, salad, bread, loader baked potato, steamed veggies, carrot cake, and at least 3 refills on her diet cola. I ordered a small salad.

Another day I was out with "Hanna-bear", who I had been friends with since kindergarten and we were at Mardi Gras in Louisiana. We had chosen one of the loudest and busiest restaurants of the night. It was Mardi Gras! We sat down and were handed menus. She let me go first and I ordered what seemed like everything on the menu! She ordered a small salad. Flashback!!

When I was with Gerry, I felt ashamed of her and upstaged her with a salad. I wanted her to see how ridiculous it was for her to have eaten that box of granola and drink that cola and then order all of that food. But I in turn had the same thing done to me by Hanna. She was embarrassed by my gluttony. So embarrassed that she not only didn't eat, but couldn't eat!

A skinny woman eats in small portions all day long. Sometimes it appears that they can eat whatever they want but many times they have a very fast metabolism which burns up their intake quickly. As we get older it's best to eat a little bit, like 4 or 5 times a day. But making sure to have that little bit be fruits, veggies, grains, lean protein and do some walking to clear your head.

It's not good to think that skipping meals will be the best way to lose weight. Skinny women or women in general who approach weight loss like that are putting their body in starvation mode. Your body will hold onto fat. Not good. Not nutritious. Get a grip!   ***

FAT BLOCKING EMBARRASSMENT

Years ago I was so desperate to lose weight I would leap at even the most ridiculous of remedies. I heard of this fat blocker pill only given by your doctor at the time. I asked my doctor about it and she gave me a prescription for it.

Low and behold it worked! You can eat what you want and your body will not absorb the fat. But....that fat that you've consumed must go somewhere. And where did it go you ask? Right into the seat onto which I sat!!!

OMG!!! It oozed out all day long. It was so much oil, like my Doctor had made a deal with Wesson or Crisco! So off to Walmart I went and had my first introduction to Adult Diapers! If I was going to take this pill, I was most certainly going to have a long love affair with Depends or Poise or whatever diapers were on sale. Finally my mom and I had something in common!!!

I felt slimy and nasty all the time. So I had to ask myself was this worth it? I came to the end of my rope when I bought the off brand sale diapers. I was dressed cute for church. Got there and sat in my seat and could feel the ooz making its way out but I felt safe...I had my diaper on and it was time for the offering. I got up to go around with my offering in my hand. I could hear paper rustling with my steps. The oil had saturated the padding and the plastic lining was no longer insulated. It was exposed to the air and had begun to rustle so if I could hear it, others could hear me as well. I walked around, right out the door and to my car. I threw those pills and those noisy diapers in the garbage!

The pills were doing exactly what they were supposed to do. I ran with my emotions and got a prescription for something that I didn't need. Those pills were $100 and I happily paid it thinking it was an easy way to "thin-hood". We waste money taking the easy route and the weight loss industry thrives on our emotions and our desperation.

As my late Aunt Helen, who was the "CoCo Chanel" of her day would say, "Diapers, my darling, are a bad look"! ***

SELF LIMITING BELIEF

Who are you? What do you like? What can you do well? While we were in our mother's womb we were being shaped mentally. I know of a woman who was told she was an accident. She should have been aborted. She should have never happened. She was a mistake. She was told this while her mother was carrying her and when she was born, she was rejected. Subsequently, she found her comfort in food. Food never rejected her. Food was sweet to her, comforting to her, always available to her. When she wanted to talk with someone, potato chips and pretzels were there. When she wanted to feel loved, candy, especially chocolate was there. That woman was me!

When you are born with rejection or you suffer the trauma of rejection, experts say that early on your beliefs about yourself begin to take root. The younger the trauma, the younger the verbal abuse the deeper the roots go and the more time they have to anchor in. Most people don't know that these roots are deep down inside and **by the time you are an adult, there is a great deal of work to undo.** The foundation has been laid over the last 30 or 50 years and it's as if it is set in cement. So the many, many years of secret repetition of "I am not good enough" have been lived out and has been such a way of life that it is nearly impossible to even recognize that it's even there. The ingrained spirit of negativity is part of your being and has been the platform for all of your bad physical and emotional wellbeing.

Some years ago my mom had a stroke and I had the time to care for her 12 hours a day, 6 days a week. Let me tell you that during that time, I had **MANY** emotions things happen to me that I absolutely did not expect nor did I know was there. But those things answered a lot of questions as to why I was an overweight child and an obese adult.

My mom would sit and watch a lot of television. Well actually she really wasn't watching it she was staring at the television and thinking. And at any given time, she would blurt out events from her life, events from her childhood, my childhood, events that I had either never known or had blocked out completely.

One day she woke up angry at my dad whom she had been married to for 25 years and has since been divorced from for more than 25 years as well. She was muttering something about having to have worked two jobs to care for my sister and I. Even though dad was paying child support and he was very much in our lives, she was still very angry that she had become a single parent. So in her muttering she blurted out that she should not have had me and that I was a mistake. I should have been aborted. I look and I act just like him. She said she should not have had any children by him. She knew when she got pregnant with me that it was a mistake. She was married four or five years before she got pregnant with me and that she should have gotten a divorce back then and should have gone on with her life and not have had any children. But she got stuck with me! What was I supposed to do with that?!?!?

When she said that, I went right back to my childhood emotionally. The rejection came back, the loneliness came back, the anger came back, the self-hatred came back, and the low self-esteem came back, and so on.... Now seven years prior to this point I had gastric bypass surgery. I was 270lbs and climbing in my weight, but then lost 145+lbs. I was happy at 125lbs, give-or-take 10 pounds. Then after my mom became ill, I became her primary caregiver and I unknowingly entered into this emotional crisis and gained nearly 70lbs. of rejection in 2 years!   I was not happy. But what was I to do?

Here I have a fragile mother who has had another stroke, who has just told me that I was never wanted and who was and still is very, very angry. Her stroke has brought her feelings about me to the surface. I really had to get a grip otherwise I would be right back where I started with my weight. And I was well on my way.

If you can imagine what great emotional pain I was in and how I could do nothing about it but listen to it every single day. What do I do? Do I walk out and go home and lick my wounds or do I stay and help her? Do I go through my own deep-level healing, work through it and continue to care for my mom? I mean who can give me that answer?

As a child, she showed me the signs that I wasn't wanted but it wasn't blatant rejection and that's not to say that she didn't love me. She loved me as much as she knew how. She was in a marriage that she didn't want to be in and had 2 children that caused her, in her mind at the time, to stay in a relationship longer than she had planned. She had rejection from her own childhood that she had never dealt with. She thought marriage would take her away from her own misery but her dream life, and dream marriage didn't pan out and she was angry about it.

This is just rejection, I haven't even discussed sexual or verbal abuse that so many people quietly suffer. Trauma of every kind stays with a child through adulthood if it is not dealt with.

Too often we are overweight because of deep rooted pain we are unaware of, nonetheless we are living it out day after day. The CDC reports that approximately one in six boys and one in four girls are sexually abused before the age of 18. In 2005, the US Department of Health and Human Services reported that 83,600 children were sexually abused. Sadly, extremely obese children, have histories of sexual abuse, which is more common than we think, and are 70 percent more likely to continue being obese into adulthood. While I'm not saying that I was sexually abused, I'm just talking about trauma in childhood period.

Being overweight is more than just eating too many potato chips and pizza. Being overweight is more than just watching endless television on the Lazy-boy 6 to 9 hours, 7 days a week. Being overweight is a domino effect from a childhood trauma, either yours or your parents. If obesity is hereditary, and if you go through your family history, you might find that someone was abused or neglected or had some sort of other trauma early in life and found comfort in food and passed that comfort down. There are certainly other factors as well but if you can dare trace it back, you will find the childhood root down in your family.

What do you do now? Where do you begin to make the change in yourself? Well, it starts from the top and ultimately runs downward. It begins in your mind. Certainly you can't help your obese relatives with their mindset, but you can help yourself! You have to have a mind change. Remember when I spoke of "deep-level healing"? Our mind is like a playground and what we choose to put in it is up to us. If we choose to limit ourselves and what we can do with our lives is purely up to us, it's not Aunt Sally's or Uncle Eugene's fault.

When I was 270lbs. I really thought that I couldn't do any better than to look good with the weight I had.

Just make sure I had the right undergarments. Then
one day I just got tired. I got tired of knee pain, back
pain, medication, sweating under my bra, breathing
hard, thighs rubbing and the threat of living a shorter
life because of my weight that I decided to do
something about it.

We self-limit because we choose to self-limit.
No one can self-limit *you for you but you!* If you mean
business like I did, I want you to begin where I began.
I believe in God and I asked God to help me get
started with cleaning out the ingrained thinking that
was put in me before I was born. Now it didn't happen
overnight or even in a few weeks but little by little
over time as I moved forward and away from that
self-limiting, self-doubting person that I was, I became
that thinner, stronger, more confident and free woman
that I longed to be. And it's a daily fight to keep clear
thoughts. In fact, in Romans 12:2 of the Bible it says,
*"So here is what I want you to do. Take your every
day, ordinary life, your sleeping, eating and going to
work, and walking around life and place it before God
as an offering. Embracing what God does for you is
the best thing you can do for him. Don't become so
well-adjusted to your culture, (way of life), that you fit
into it without even thinking. Instead, fix your
attention on God. You'll be changed from the inside
out. Readily recognize what He wants from you, and
quickly respond to it. Unlike the culture around you,
always dragging you down to its level of immaturity,
God brings the best out of you, develops well-formed
maturity in you."*

As I said, I am still developing myself and what I have
found is that it is a never, ever ending process. The
older you get, the more you realize you have so much
to learn. Man, if I had not had God with me when my
mom said those things to me, I would have blacked

out! It was devastating enough with God so I can't even imagine how I would have dealt with that information without God! You might say that my Mom didn't mean the things that she said and that may be true in part. I don't fault her, I have learned to guard my own heart. On a good day she and I still have really good conversations and we laugh and joke. But there has always been this undertone of deep, deep anger and frustration that she has to admit she holds. I am only telling you this because I want you to recognize it in yourself, if I am speaking to you, and you really feel this, I want you to get somewhere and get help dealing with that hurtful part of your past. It truly stays with you **all of your life** if you don't get the help that you need.

Certainly I went through all of the anger and disappointment and things that I mentioned and began to gain my weight back, *but when I began to get a grip, and forgive, I began to go through that deeper healing with God and cry it out.* Understand, your process might not be like mine but nonetheless, it will be a process that you alone must go through. And the only way to go through it is to *go through it.* And when you get through it is when the healing process of the traumas that you have suffered, whenever you suffered them, will begin to finally start you on your process of losing weight. It may take 6 months, a year or 2 years, that doesn't matter but it will begin. This is one of your personal steps that makes your weight lose your own process and not a cookie cutter program. When you get through this part, you will feel like you can take on every single thing in the world because you took the bull by the horns and ran him into the ground yourself!!!!

Years later as life would have it, I worked for Jenny Craig. I was the Program Director, the one who brought the business or the clientele to the center. I was also the one who was responsible for the sales and commissions of my fellow employees. In short, we all got paid because I made the major sales.

It was on my shoulders to get the clients or customers to purchase the largest program they could as well as buy up as much of that company's food products. My point is this, every customer that came in got the same program, the same cuisine, whether it be the Imitation Strawberry, Blueberry or Chocolate Cheesecake Desserts or the Chicken flavored Tofu Pot-sticker dinners...yuck! Nothing was tailor-made for them. They taught us a power-point presentation and just how to pitch it to get that sale. And it didn't really matter if the customer gained or lost weight. What mattered was that they spent money, a lot of money on anything from that company!

I could not tell you the amount of women as well as men who came into my office who confessed some kind of trauma, whether it was sexual, mental or emotional abuse from their childhood, but one after another they would come in and sit and cry and tell me that they absolutely could not lose their weight. They have tried everything and now they have come here for me to help them.

This we were not trained on. We were not given the okay to hold their hand and talk out their various abuse issues. We were not mental health counselors and I understood that, however ***don't sell weight loss if you really cannot help the person with weight loss!***

We were only trained how to get money from them... NO MATTER WHAT! Never mind they had a late car note or mortgage payment due, corporate would come in monthly and drill us on pressing the client for that

Life Program Membership. So what if they had their kids school tuition due, corporate told me that my job was on the line if I didn't sell enough life program memberships which at the time were in upwards of $500 plus the weekly cost of THEIR food. Certainly I could sell them $20 starter programs along with the weekly meals but that was not the goal.

Sadly, I was fired after a year because my conscience wouldn't allow me to overlook their abuse issues, their financial issues and take their money for the sake of the company. The stress of it all was so great that I ended up in the hospital with what appeared to be either a mild heart attack or a severe stress attack. I just know that my heart was aching so severely from the pain of these clients and the pressure of this company. They failed to see that obese people have far greater issues than just weight and using their vulnerability to take their money was just wrong for me and it still is. If you are going to help someone in any capacity, help them and along with helping them, you should be teaching them how to help themselves because you will not always be there.

So here you are today with your weight issues….still! I am telling you that you have to break through your emotional trauma for yourself so that you can customize your own plan for yourself. No one else cares about your weight lose as much as you do. I can give you every bit of my information and even hold your hand but I am not on the inside of you. You are there on the inside, in the middle of the night questioning yourself, angry with yourself, frustrated with yourself.

In the quietness and secrecy of your own mind you speak to yourself every day. Maybe you rehearse those past traumas in your mind every night. Perhaps there were no initial trauma or you cannot remember them. But what are you saying to yourself? There was a cartoon that I use to watch as a child every Christmas called, "Chris Cringle," and in the cartoon there was a boy who sang a song called, "Put One Foot In Front of the Other." The song goes on to say that, *"Soon you will be walking across the floor, with one foot in front of the other, soon you'll be walking out of the door!"* I may have gotten the name of the cartoon wrong and even the name of the song, but the attitude of the song is what I'm getting at. I want you to put one foot in front of the other so that you can walk across that floor and then put one foot in front of the other so that you can walk right out that FAT door!   ***

<u>IS IT ME?</u>

Let's get a little technical right here. I mentioned earlier that obesity might have come from your family line. Let us discuss what is in your direct control, what is in your indirect control and what is out of your control that has brought you to this point in your life. Even though it may have been in your family line, you may have *aided the condition of obesity.*

1.   **<u>DIRECT CONTROL</u>**

What are your everyday decisions? Do you eat at every fast-food restaurant that you pass? Do you reward yourself for a job well done or pig out because of a horrible job done for the day? **I did!**

What are your everyday actions? Do you eat out more than you should? Is it a sit-down joint or a drive through thing? Do you eat out because you don't want to cook or can't cook? Do you eat out because it's easier to do so and you don't want to make the effort or is your life too busy and you can't get organized? **I did!**

You are directly living in the choices that you have made. That burger and fries or those ribs with the loaded baked potato and the cake have brought you right to this very point. Even the salad and all the dressing with the soda have done it as well. Because you are doing more than just the salad, more than just the fast-food joint on Thursdays, it's the chips at the gas station and the cupcake after church and the three Pepsi's at work and the pizza with the girls on Saturday and the sitting and sitting and above all, ***it's your attitude about yourself.***

If you are in a community where there is emphasis on walking, biking, hiking and other outdoor activities, chances are you will engage in these activities. Likewise, if everything and everyone around you are eating fast foods, sitting, partying, drinking, you will indulge and often. **It's our need to be included in the masses.** But what you must recognize are the masses right for me? You have to be honest with what you are doing so that you can get started. *Self-denial will keep you either on this page or tell you to close this book.* However, truth and self-discovery will have you continue onto the following pages. Shall we continue?

2.   **<u>INDIRECT CONTROL</u>**

Your environment has a great deal to do with your weight as well. Your genes are up to 70% responsible for your body's weight. They determine how heavy your body wants to be. In actuality, your genes are your body's "Set Point". But...*your genes are not set in stone.....*You can certainly work around them, much like working around reading the cliffs-notes instead of reading the entire book when you were in school! It may or may not be a good thing. It depends on how you are getting around them.

Getting around your Set Points the wrong way involves doing things such as:

•	**Appetite Suppressants.** They aid in making you feel full, these suppressants are products that use various combinations of drugs to promote weight loss by manipulating hormonal and chemical processes in the body that control hunger pangs and the sense of feeling full or satiated. The problem with these drugs are that they *synthetically fool your brain* to think you are full but when you get off of them , you balloon up more often worse than when you started!

•	**Diet Pills or Lipase Inhibitors**. They work by stopping your body from being able to absorb and digest excessive amounts of fat in the food you eat on a regular basis, like my fat pills. Though this method of weight loss may be right for some and sound like it will do all of the work for you, as with all drugs, it comes with pro's and con's.

Pros: Lipase inhibitors are meant to block the absorption of fats in the food that you eat, and so they aid in losing weight by stopping your body from being able to take in many fats you may be eating. Certain diet pills have been shown to reduce blood pressure. It has also been seen that certain lipase inhibitors can help prevent the onset of type 2 diabetes. Whether these two side effects are due to the medications themselves or the resulting weight loss is unknown.

Cons: Not only do lipase inhibitors block the absorption of fat, but they can also stop your body from being able to digest certain vitamins. They have been known to cause excessive gas, incontinence, urgent bowel movements and oily spotting. A significant number of those who use lipase inhibitors and then stop will regain the weight they had lost during the time they were not taking the medications.

- **Weight Loss Surgery:** This alters your body's way of processing food and getting around your body's Set Point to become obese. Just how weight loss surgery reduces weight is through Gastro-intestinal surgery for the obese, which is also called bariatric surgery. It alters the digestive process so as to achieve rapid weight loss. You must ***painfully go against*** the surgery to gain your weight back....and so many people painfully do!

- **Commercial Programs:** The weight-loss industry sells hope to desperate people every minute of every day. Americans spend more than $40 billion a year on weight-loss programs and weight loss products. They answer the enticement to "lose 20 pounds for just $20 plus the cost of food".

According to a recent study reported most people who participate in weight-loss programs "regain about one-third of the weight lost during the first year and are typically back to baseline in three to five years." But you didn't need to be a rocket scientist to have discovered that. *Celeb's who are paid millions, are given free food from the weight loss companies, their own special trainers and sign contracts to get thin and stay thin and help that selected company look good for the next year.* Remember, I said these Celebrities get paid MILLIONS to help a company look spectacular and their process for losing weight look simple! But sometimes these high-paid celebrities fall back into comfortable habits and regain their weight, and with all of the help and support literally given to them, they still can't, don't or won't honor their contract, so why would it be any different for the rest of us?

Someone said plain and simply, *"Here's why we overeat: Food tastes good, so we eat lots of it. Here's why we gain weight: We take in more calories than we burn off. Here's the only way to maintain weight loss: Eat less and exercise more for the rest of your life."* Ugh!!!! Isn't it just easier to buy willpower in the form of a weight loss program or pill or buy a weight loss program in the form of a willpower pill?! Either way you must make a choice and work at it. The mind must change before the body can change! ***

<u>Diets Do Not Work At All.</u>

There's no doubt about it: Diets don't work for most Americans. It's easy to blame the diets, but it's more accurate to blame the dieters.

We are a *"Right Now" society and want immediate gratification. The chore of grinding out a weight loss plan can be frustrating. We can't quickly back up a forward growing belly or speed up a two-hour cardio workout in the gym, but we want it and we want it in 10 minutes! "Americans are looking for that silver bullet,"* says Keri Gans, a registered dietician and national spokesperson for the American Dietetic Assn. *"But they won't change their behavior. That's where the fault lies."*

Many diet programs market themselves as lifestyle choices, rather than silver bullets even though that's what they want you to think they are. The infamous South Beach Diet and Atkins Diet wants their followers to live a life based on their limited, controlled regimen. Let's be real. You will once again spend the money on their plan because it sounds fabulous but after falling off, will put the plan in "Drawer 13!" These plans are not intended for real life. None of them are.

The $40+ billion Americans spend on diet plans each year is a weighty amount, for sure. But those billions represent aspirations rather than effort. ***Dieters who want to fit into thinner jeans for more than a few months or years need to find a plan that will fit into their REAL LIFE lifestyle.*** If we're wasting billions of dollars on fruitless diets, it's likely the fault lies not just with Jenny or even Atkins but with ourselves as well.

If we stop "feeding" into these programs that don't work, and if we are not going to work them 100%, they will stop growing!

3.   **<u>OUT OF YOUR CONTROL</u>**

- **Obesity Virus**

This might be outrageous but there is a virus that causes obesity! The obesity virus increases the amount that your fat cells can hold and speeds up the rate at which they mature. Although it can be "caught" from other people, not everyone who has it is obese or even overweight. One study found that about 30% of obese people and 11% of lean people have the virus in their system.

Often, educated physicians will say, "Obesity is a disease," but not many people believe it. The government and insurance companies do not want to admit that obesity is a disease because then they would have to cover treatment as they do for other diseases. Even a large portion of healthcare professionals who treat obesity do not necessarily think of obesity as a disease. This may be because the treatments they provide are based on obesity being a behavioral problem that can only be treated by changing behaviors, such as dietary, exercise habits and lifestyle. Just like you may catch the common cold virus, one-third of people affected by obesity have been infected and multiple investigators around the world have started to work on this virus!

From this chapter, I hope you have learned plenty. It is my hopes that you will see that there is so much more to your weight than just putting aside your burger and fries and having surgery or spending money on another plan. A great deal of intimate thought should go into what, when, how and why you are going to reshape your body and your life. It can absolutely be done and only you can do it. **However, it takes concentrated and deliberate architectural planning, in a sense, to reconstruct a new monument called YOU!**   ***

OMAR THE TENT MAKER

My father use to tease me about my weight in all sorts of subtle ways all of my life. When I was in my 20's and 30's, I was at the height of my weight issues, and he would use the phrase, "Where did you get that dress from, Omar?" At the time, I didn't know who Omar was, nor did I get the joke. When I'd look at him with that blank, "don't–get-the-joke" look, he'd just crack his side laughing at me. He was referring to the amount of fabric needed to make the dress or blouse I might have been wearing at the time. He didn't mean to hurt my feelings that was just his way.

Once I understood the joke, it use to hurt my feelings something awful but he would never see it. I would just swallow it down along with another fork full of something! The anxiety was all consuming because it was a statement and an unspoken acknowledgement that I was fat and everyone in my family could see it but would never dare say it....just him. So every Christmas, Easter, Thanksgiving and family gathering,

I'd "gulp", ring the doorbell and enter in with a smile and wait for Omar to greet me!

My sister was the skinny one, my mom was the beautiful one, and dad was the smart one so quite naturally I rationalized in my head that I had to be the fat one. My husband would do what he could to comfort me but when you are inside the skin of a fat person, there are **no right words of comfort.** Really the more you try to comfort a fat person with nice words the more that person turns to food. Food is the comfort. That's the soft place to fall....and fall often! I fell nearly 300 times!!

We've talked about this in a previous chapter, it's estimated that most overweight people have been abused either verbally, sexually or emotional early in their lives and have turned to food for their source of comfort and support. Food was my comfort for most of my life. When I decided to break from that traumatic cycle by whatever means necessary, the healing could begin. That doesn't mean it was easy. It means it was worth it!

To get from one place in a room to the next, a skinny woman merely walks from here to there. *A fat person, instinctively has learned to scan the room to see the safest and least embarrassing and most inconspicuous route to take to get to the easiest available seat.* I know this because I have done both. The first time I caught myself panning the room I had to ask myself, "What the heck was I doing?" I was looking for the least embarrassing route to take so that I wouldn't knock over a chair or tip a table or bump a kid in the head with my purse or my hip...or worse, my purse <u>on</u> my hip! We all have seen it!

Clever maneuvering is a way of life for a fat person. That's one of the many reasons why fat people are so exhausted and sweaty when they sit down. *They have been in mental as well as physical traffic all day every day!* Skinny people just don't have to do that or even think about it, they just live. Heavy people unconsciously worry about the furniture breaking underneath them or the arms of the chair popping off from the pressure of their hips. And after a while the worry becomes a way of life.

We all have seen very heavy women who can flawlessly apply their makeup and do their hair and when it's all said and done, they are extremely breathtaking from their shoes to their dress and jewelry to their perfect face and hair. But inside they are not happy.

I met a woman who was tall, beautiful, and full of style, grace and glamour. Her speech, her attire and every jewel on her neckline was just so on point. Upon entering her home I was knocked out by the soft woodsy scented candles she had burning. Her home was like something out of Martha Stewart. Every room was creatively colorful, relaxing and inviting with very expensive pieces of artwork placed just right, family pictures and other home goods placed in just the right spots. She was in fact the granddaughter of a prominent national black figure and she was very, very proud of who she was.

She invited me to go into her lower level which was where we were to spend our time discussing her weight dilemmas. Holy Moses! Her lower level was a "Girl Cave" to die for!!! Floor to ceiling and wall to wall flat screen, more beautiful pictures of her famous family on ALL of the walls. A chocolate circular sectional and every piece of exercise equipment you could name. Everything in yellows, browns and pinks if you can imagine!

SKINNY WOMEN ARE NOT CREATED EQUAL

As we sat down and began to talk, she started to cry almost instantly. I held her hand and said nothing but allowed her to say and do what she needed to. She said with all of this fabulous house, her famous name, and her personal accomplishments, all she saw in the mirror was a fat girl. She was married and had a daughter but the marriage didn't last because she was too fat. She said she was nearing 400lbs. but that's not the sad part. She had the stomach surgery and was not even 300lbs. when she had it. She bought things and dressed up and puts on a ton of make up to cover up how ugly she felt inside. And with that she just cried and cried.

All I heard inside my heart for her was abandonment. If she were pretty enough her father would not have left her. If she were skinny enough her husband would not have left her. So I asked her where was her husband and her father? She said they both were gone and she didn't know. She had so much work to do on the inside before she could ever begin the lose weight and keep it off.

I told her to take a deep breath. What are the facts? Let me ask you, what are your facts? Her father is gone from her life. Her husband is gone from her life. You stop growing at the point of the hurt and with that being the case, if her father left her at 7, although she might have been 52, when we began to talk about abandonment and she broke down and began to cry about her father, she was a 7 year old all over again. Even when her husband left her, she turned into that little girl looking for daddy and took another bite of that Almond Joy Candy bar!

See it, say it, confess that it happened, cry over it and then you must figure out how to move on from it. Otherwise you will be stuck for years in it. **DO NOT REHEARSE THE HURT.** In other words, if this woman's husband left her for another woman, she can't continue to say over and over like the little girl in the movie "Jurassic Park", "He left us, he left us!!!!" She could be chained to him and all of those memories of when he left and then what a great life they could have had. Meanwhile he has gone on with his life and she is 400lb of rehearsed pain. You have to get on with your own life and you can't if you are chained.

She needs to get a life....YOU NEED TO GET A LIFE. It is time for you to rediscover yourself. Reinvent yourself. Reconstruct a new monument of YOU!!! Change yourself. **The best revenge is to develop yourself. Make yourself your own project. Concentrate on you.** If you need to find a new church or a new set of friends or build a new wardrobe or get a new hair color, then do that. You are going to do all of this while you now begin to lose your weight. It takes time but time is going to pass anyway. My Pastor said in Service the other day and I'd like you to write this down,   **"TIME TAKES TIME."** Put the focus on you and not on anyone else. That's not to say that you should become self-centered, but your rediscovery is not someone else's job. Your happiness is not someone else's responsibility. *The making of you is not for someone else to do. This is solely your job.* What you haven't done or what the past has done to you is not your focus. Focus on you and your future you, not on your past traumas. If you have children, focus on rebuilding your life with them. If you don't have children, get a bird or a puppy or a stuffed bear or even a fake baby. Do this for yourself today so that your future self will thank you tomorrow.

It's a brand new day and it's going to be a brand new you!!   ***

STANDING IN FRONT OF THE CLOSET

Every single Sunday morning it was the same routine, my husband would get up and stumble down the hall into the boys' rooms and say, "Rise and shine, shine and rise, time to get up, let's open our eyes. Let's go, let's go, let's go!" Then everyone would be up and spinning around the bathroom getting ready for Morning Worship Service.

I, on the other hand, would be crying in my closet. I put off selecting my outfit until the very last of the last minute because I could not connect with any item hanging there. Everything was a tent in every color of the spectrum and I was tired of them. Orange tents with red spots, brown tents with white piping, blue tents with gold buttons, you name it I had it.

I had the clothes for my 4 little boys and my baby girl ready the night before. My husband would do the guy stuff and I would take care of my daughter after I got myself together. However, every Sunday getting myself together was as grievous for me as digging a hole would probably be for Snow White! I hated what I had to choose from and I hated my size 26 Woman's on a 5ft high medium frame which was just awful. My body structure made it worse; no butt to speak of, no hips, a short waist and 44-ff boobs made me look like I was always carrying a watermelon! Ooh, but I had a great face and personality, when I wasn't crying at is!!!

My husband just didn't know how to console me. The more he spoke, the more I cried. I could not wait for Sunday to leave. Monday through Saturday was bearable, but Sunday was just awful day after week after month after year for 35 years. You would have

thought I'd gotten used to it but I hadn't. I learned to smile in public and wail in private. I was simply...
<u>MISERABLE!</u>

What I eventually learned was *if you really, really loath a thing about your life, only you can change it.* Not your mother, nor your girlfriend, definitely not your husband or anyone that you love or says they love you. You have to do it for yourself and not for anyone else. If they leave your life....are you going to stop or keep going? And you can't blame anyone from your past for your present weight. You are grown now. Take responsibility, no matter how painful, and YOU MAKE THE CHANGE.

You have to figure it out for yourself and then draw out the roadmap that you are going to follow. You may have to make changes once you get out there on that open road but the point is that you are finally getting out there!

I wailed, cried, and complained until I couldn't wail, cry or complain any more. I couldn't stand to hear myself another minute. I would walk a mile every day, (exercise alone is not enough by the way), and I'd look to the sky and ask God to show me how to change myself. There had to be a way for me to reinvent me. You see 20-25 years ago, I had so very little knowledge about weight loss surgery. It was fairly new and something that only movie stars and wealthy people did. I didn't know of anyone who had done such a thing. Also to this point every diet that I had tried, failed me. I had little faith in anything diet. God had to split the sky and do something else for me because to this point nothing seemed to work.

If I could figure out a plan and then begin walking out this plan, there was going to be no way I was going to be stopped. I didn't care how long it took me. I had been miserable for far too darn long. I was in a size 28 Woman's and that was even more depressing! When the buttons on your 26 Woman's shirt are pulling, you gotta stop what you are doing and do something else! That's where I was. I had to do something else. I was tired of crying in the closet, I was tired of my buttons pulling, I was tired of all the diets and all the wailing, I had to put together a plan...my own plan. I had to do something. What I was sure of was... SOMETHING WAS OUT THERE LOOKING FOR ME THAT WOULD WORK! Whenever I get my hands on it, there would be no going back. I just didn't know what that was but I was looking. ***

2 LIFE TIME MEMBERSHIPS

Walking, or should I say waddling through Wal-Mart, I made the decision to become the spokesperson for "Slim-fast" so I purchased every item that they had on the shelves and in every flavor.

Strawberry, Vanilla and Chocolate canned shakes and breakfast bars. Well, I lasted one whole week in a row! I'm sure I was not supposed to be absolutely starving on their products. A breakfast bar in the morning, a shake at mid-day, a salad for lunch, another shake at mid-afternoon and a good sensible dinner. But somewhere in there I was going nuts! I was starving and shaking and incredibly tired. No fault of that company, I just figured it was not the right one for me. They didn't give me the nutrition that I needed. They were starving me by my permission so I couldn't complain about it. I didn't want to waste all that I had purchased so I added vitamins and fruit to the routine. Aaah...it helped some but not enough to stop me from shaking. I concluded that I was getting too much of one thing and not enough of something else. So it was time to move onto plan #2!

I had already tried Jenny and she didn't seem to work for me and now that I am home and not working, I am way too far from the Center that I started with, (I didn't yet know that they had closed), and I wasn't going to haul it out there twice a week to make any meeting just to satisfy my lifetime membership.

I was out running errands and stumbled across a Jenny around my house. Aha!!!!! And being desperate I did what any housewife would do without thinking, I went in and let them talk me into <u>another</u> "Life-Time Membership"!

They could not find me in their system. Well what good is a membership of that length if you are not going to keep up with it? So I paid another $500 bucks, plus I purchased a weeks' worth of Jenny food. Once home I remembered receiving a packet of information at the first enrollment. The questions was where did I put it? So I began looking for it. Over the course of a few months I found the package that proved that I had a previous membership, only now *I owned 2 Lifetime Memberships.* I brought in the proof and although they acknowledged it, they could do nothing about it other than honor the new one when the first one runs out!!! LIFE TIME.....Duh!!!

Years later I became an employee of the company. It was so hard to separate myself from being in the shoes of each client that I had. I would remember like it was still happening when I was sitting in the same seat, crying my eyes out, wanting the counselor to just help me to become like the skinny woman on the poster on the wall. It didn't even matter at the time that the counselor, whose name was Val, had never been fat a darn day in her life, she could not help me. I didn't understand that then.

Being an employee gave me so much insight into the fact that all Val wanted to do was get her commission at the end of the day. She used my emotions and sold me as much as she could. If she could use my emotions against me, she could "up" her check! She didn't care about me, really. It was about her children, her mortgage and her car note at the end of the day. No fault of hers, that's how she was trained. She needed to make money.

That's why I was fired. I couldn't ride on the emotions of my clients no matter how far behind my mortgage was or how much on the line my job was. The Training Supervisors from corporate, gave me a deadline to have so many "lifetimes" sold or say "good bye" to my job. It was so much more important to me that my clients know how much I cared about them than for them to care how much I knew about the Jenny System, Products and food. On my birthday, July 16th, was my last day of work. They asked me to say "good bye". I actually went to the hospital from work with what was a severe stress attack. At the time, though I thought it was a heart attack. The stress to perform and take advantage of people was ridiculous.

I learned so much while in that camp. Among the things that I learned was even more compassion for people. You never know where people have come from. They will always tell you one thing so that they can get through their day, but in reality their life has had many traumatic episodes. ***

BAD DOCTOR

Weight was a daily issue. As much as I would render that inner negative conversation dead, something would happen that would remind me that I am just too big. Whether it was not fitting in the seat in the theater or looking at what I was actually eating in a restaurant, the truth is the truth. You can dress it down or ignore it if you like but it is always there.

My husband and I went on a cruise and I was determined to enjoy myself. I was not going to make my weight an issue. My husband loved me just the way that I was and that was going to be that. I got my braids put in my hair, bought a new swim suit, with a cover up, of course, and had purchased the cutest island outfits for the week.

On the deck of the boat there was a waterslide and my husband was daring enough to try it. "Swoosh," he went down and splashed into the pool. So, I decided to give it a try. It was hot as we headed towards the island of Antigua and everybody was out and about on deck.

I was brave enough to take off my cover-up and with my husband's encouragement I headed up the steps of the waterslide. At the top the attendant told me to lay down on my back and cross my arms over my chest and the water will take me right down. So that's what I did. I gave my husband the thumbs up and laid down.

Now, after a second or two I could not feel any water taking me down. However, I could feel it rushing around my ears and then spilling over the top of me! A kid yells out, "Hey, what's taking so long?!" Ooh man.....the sheer embarrassment of being stuck on that slide was more than I could handle! My husband was at the bottom helpless and there was a long line forming behind me.

I did my best to scoot myself down but I was burning my thighs on the sides of the slide. Ooh No! I was doing my best not to cry and cover it all up with a nervous laugh as the kids behind me were screaming for me to go down and the attendant saw that I was in distress. He was yelling at me to lay sideways so that the water could take me down. Certainly it ruined the rest of the day and a great deal of the rest of vacation. I got stuck on a waterslide!! I got stuck on a waterslide!! I rehearsed that event the entire vacation. No matter how hard I tried to shake that incident off, how could it not affect me?

Too often I'd run into women who would say to me, "Girl I don't put that much energy into my weight like that. Just as long as I look good in my clothes!" However, when you have pain in your knees, and you can't run around with your children, or your breathing is labored because you went up 4 steps, or you can't control your embarrassing sweating or even situations like I just mentioned, or worse, you can't buckle your gorgeous shoes and the center of your jeans disintegrate after only a few wears, you gotta know you have to do something about your weight. As for putting energy into the fat suit you wear beautifully every day, IT IS NOT OKAY!

You can fool many people but you cannot fool yourself. This I found out to be painfully true. Even though I did my absolute best to look smashing in everything...every tent or sometimes every suit I wore, and was colorful and made sure I had room in my clothing and matched everything up with the right accessories, inside I was SCREAMING!!!! I tried Jenny and everybody else, but.... I was tired of the war.

I had heard of weight loss surgery but was too afraid to even look into it. When I got off that plane following that business meeting I was absolutely done with myself! I promised myself that I would never go through that private humiliation again.

After I got home and relaxed myself, I began surfing the internet to school myself on weight loss surgery. Ooh man, there was far too much for me to pick through. So I left it alone and sulked for a few weeks about how pitiful my life was.

One fine Sunday morning I ran into Joanie, a longtime friend who had just had the surgery and was telling me about her ordeal. She happened to have her doctor's business card in her purse and gave it to me. That started the ball rolling; so now I had a direction to follow.

I got on my computer and read everything I could on her doctor, on his background, on the hospital he worked out of and everything else that I could find on him. I didn't really care how the procedure was done as much as how it was going to be paid for so I skimmed over the procedure part and went onto the insurance part.

That's when I felt the floor cave in! Everything seemed to be as right as rain. The doctor had a perfect record, the hospital was at the top of their medical game for the best bariatric surgery unit and the most efficient team in the Midwest but my insurance was not accepted. Ugh!!!! So I closed up my computer and went into my pillow and cried!

Somewhere in my childhood I heard that there was more than one way to 'skin a cat'. It was coming up on November and I desperately wanted to start off the New Year with a new project, "ME"! I called another hospital in the city that was also known for its bariatric surgery. I spoke with the nurse and asked a lot of questions. They took my insurance...Yeah!!!!! Immediately I made my appointment for the coming February 10, 2002. I was HAPPY!

November came and went and so did December and January. About the 3rd or 4th of February I called and asked them why hadn't I received a phone call for any blood work or anything to get me ready for the surgery. The nurse handed the phone to the doctor who just happened to be standing next to her at the time. This is what he said to me, ***"It is totally up to you to get all the necessary lab work, psychological work and nutritional education. I just do the surgery!"*** I said to him that I had no idea what I would need done before surgery. He in turn said to me, ***"That's not my problem, I just do the surgery."***

With that I cancelled my surgery with lightning speed and returned to my pillow! I was desperate, not crazy! ***

HOPE, IF YOU CAN STAND IT

So with that great let down I was back at square one. How was I going to get this surgery thing done? Forget 'skinning the cat,' I set it free! Maybe I will have to return to Jenny….a frightening thought, but nonetheless it was a fast approaching reality if I wanted to lose weight, or so I thought.

I thought I had no options. The products sold on the Superstore shelves never worked. The fat doctor stuff had me chasing my tail, Jenny took my money twice and the prescription crap had me squirting oil! What was I to do? My insurance was not accepted and in 2003 the surgery costs for such was in the clouds. I was raising 5 hefty children, owned a home, excuse me…I had a mortgage, had 2 cars, again…excuse me, car notes, leather furniture, large screen television, a dog, 2 cats, 40 fish and buttons popping off my approaching size 28w wardrobe! I thought I had it going on but I was absolutely suffering inside. I had to get something done.

In my depression I sat and decided to revisit the bariatric sites I was given by my friend, Joanie. It was now after the first of the year and there were all new before and after pictures posted on the doctor's site. This of course made me feel "worser"..., jealous even. I WANTED ME TO BE IN THOSE PICTURES!!!!!! So in this fat body I thought I was confined. I either had to decide to deal with it for another 40 years or find a new cat to skin!

While on the computer, I asked my husband to go out to retrieve the mail and he came back with a packet of information from his place of employment. This packet included the new health insurance information for the New Year that he had chosen without my knowledge. At some point in my weakened and depressed state, God had pity on me and lined up all the ducks, pretty-like, in a row. The Bible is true, God is so faithful and Jesus really is Lord! It turned out that the very insurance that I needed, the very insurance that my friend, Joanie's doctor accepted, was the same insurance that my dear husband had chosen in the New Year. I had not ever discussed those details with him but he was moved to change insurances. For whatever the reason was, I was soo thankful!!!!! So much so that I called and got an appointment as quick as I could. Bye-bye kitty cat!!!   ***

GOOD DOCTOR

Ooh Wee... I was bouncing around the house.... literally.... waiting for my appointment. The very first consultation was free so that right there was a plus. If I didn't like what I heard I was under no obligation to pay anything.

SKINNY WOMEN ARE NOT CREATED EQUAL

As I sat in the waiting room, I noticed it was laced with Dr. Jerry's many Chicago accomplishments and Bariatric organizations he was affiliated with. There were many pamphlets available for me to read but to my surprise, there were also very large chairs all the way around the room. I don't know why that was surprising to me but it was. Everyone who comes in to see Dr. Jerry has a weight problem so why wouldn't the chairs be extra-large?

Anyway, after I filled out all of the necessary paperwork, my name was called and I happily followed the nurse and went in. She took my weight and then invited me to have a seat in the examining room and wait for Dr. Jerry. He came in moments later and he was very nice, very pleasant and very doctor-ish in sort of an "Alan Alda" from M.A.S.H. kind of way! He began to explain every single thing about the process of before, during and after surgery to me.

First he was very encouraging. He took my official weight which was an obscene, 267lbs., the same weight as the new Heavy-weight boxing contender of the world, at the time...another Ugh! Then he explained to me what my BMI, my Body Mass Index was. Based on your weight, this is a measure of body fat based on height and weight that applies to adult men and women. If I am more than a measurement of 30 based on my 5ft., 2in, frame, then I am obese. Well I was considered "Super-Obese. I had a BMI something like 48.

Then he began to tell me about the hospital and his team. He was adamant in telling me that their Bariatric Surgery Center is dedicated to safely and effectively treating patients who are 100 pounds or more over their ideal body weight. They understand the pain of diet and exercise failures, and after so long, people just lose hope that they can ever lose their weight. I was crying and *I was sold!!!*

He said that they strive to reduce the problems related to obesity with a team of specialists. Then he went onto tell me that his team consists of bariatric surgeons, a support staff which includes nutritionists, exercise therapists, psychologists and the list goes on. I didn't even get in the door with that "Bad doctor!"

And the moral of this story is, if you can't get an appointment with a doctor and he doesn't talk about a team of people that will support you from start to finish, HE should be finished!

I happened to visit my doctor's website and here is some of his bedside manner-isms that I found to be true from my experience: **"Our specialized team has a vast experience in treating obesity.... In fact, we've been rated** *Bariatric Surgery Center of Excellence* **based on quality and overall excellence. And, with comprehensive consultation, counseling, support and long-term follow-up, our team brings their expertise together to give you the best options in one place."**

My entire process was so magnificent, that I'd do it *one hundred times over again* because of the excellent care I received. Let me say that I only received excellent care because I did my research and figured out what questions to ask, what to look for and what kind of experienced doctor I was going to be working with.

When I began this journey, I had absolutely no idea and the other doctor knew that I was not prepared, thus he was prepared to get as much from my insurance company or my pocket as he could!

SKINNY WOMEN ARE NOT CREATED EQUAL

My doctor's site also shares that, **"...the Center is focused on reducing the pain of surgery as much as possible."** And this is very true in my case. They specialize in minimally invasive laparoscopic techniques including Roux-en-Y Gastric Bypass Surgery, which is what I had, and the Lap-Band® Adjustable Gastric Band. These are the two most popular types of surgery you want to know and do your own research on when you are looking for a doctor. By the way, it's been 15 years and not only does he remember me, I can call or go in for any health or stomach related issue and he will gladly see me

"Good treatment is important in all areas of our center, not just the operating room. Our staff sees every patient as an individual. Your treatment will be based on many factors and considered carefully. Overcoming obesity requires changing your lifestyle, and we're here to make sure we take every step <u>with you</u> and provide as much information as needed." And it's for these reasons that I had *thee* best experience.

However, I have come across far too many people who just literally lay down and say, "Please cut me open and make me skinny!" Some of these people, sad to say, have had horrible and even fatal outcomes. But there is a simple rule of thumb. <u>If you would not just sit back and open your mouth and pour any kind of medicine down your throat, don't allow any doctor to rearrange your insides just because he says he can do it!</u> Be proactive and do your own research so when you walk in the door, and hop up on that table for your very first exam, there are no surprises!   ***

SURGERY DECISION

I made the decision to have weight-loss surgery literally before I walked into Dr. Jerry's office. Once I had been in his office and he solidified my decision by explaining to me the differences and we could agree on which one was best for me, I then could take all of the information back to my own regular doctor for submission to my health insurance company and she could begin the lengthy process of preparing me for surgery.

I thought it was going to be cut and dry, however it definitely was not. It was going to take at least 9 to 10 months of me doing a bit of work on my part to prove that I was not only serious, but committed to this vast change. And for Dr. Jerry and his staff to do all of the testing that they needed to do for this surgery to be successful, I had to put some of my own "skin in the game" too!

My personal doctor, Dr. Kay got busy and submitted everything necessary to my insurance company, then after taking my vitals she looked me square in the eyes and told me this is not a simple matter. This is major surgery. The surgery that I had chosen, which was the Gastric Bypass, was permanent and there was no going back. I had to cooperate with my own decision and in doing so, my very first step was to lose 10 pounds on my own. She said that this would help me get through the procedure more comfortably. Any weight lost going into this type of surgery is always better than any weight gained.

Weight-loss surgeries make changes to your digestive system to help you lose weight by limiting how much you can eat or by reducing the absorption of nutrients, or both. These surgeries are done when diet programs and exercise haven't worked or when you have serious health problems because of your weight.

There are many types of weight-loss surgeries, known collectively as bariatric surgery. Gastric bypass is one of the most common types of bariatric surgery in the United States and the one that I settled on. Many surgeons prefer gastric bypass surgery because it generally has fewer complications than do other weight-loss surgeries.

Weight-loss surgery is done to help you lose excess weight and reduce your risk of potentially life-threatening weight-related health problems, including:

•Gastro-esophageal reflux disease

•Heart disease

•High blood pressure

•Severe sleep apnea

•Type 2 diabetes

•Stroke

Weight-loss surgeries are typically done only AFTER you've tried to lose weight by improving your diet and exercise habits as mapped out by your doctor after you have begun your journey towards your surgery. Your Doctor need to document your efforts.

In general, weight-loss surgeries could be an option for you if:

•Your body mass index (BMI) is 40 or higher (extreme obesity)....which mine was!

•Your BMI is 35 to 39.9 (obesity), AND you have a serious weight-related health problem, such as type 2 diabetes, high blood pressure or severe sleep apnea....which I was on my way to having all of these!

In some cases, you may qualify for certain types of weight-loss surgery if your BMI is 30 to 34 and you have serious weight-related health problems. Do your research and talk with your doctor!

Classification	**BMI**
Underweight	19 or less
Ideal BMI	19 – 24.9
Overweight	25 – 29.9
Obese	30 and higher
Severely Obese	35 and higher
Morbidly Obese	40 and higher
Super Obese	50 and higher

Ask your Doctor what your BMI is or go online to find your BMI Classification. ***

WHAT IS IT EXACTLY?

Gastric bypass isn't for everyone who is severely overweight. You may need to meet certain medical guidelines to qualify for weight-loss surgery. If you have a thorough doctor, they should put you through an extensive screening process to see if you qualify. You must also be willing, willing and, "WILLING" to make permanent changes to lead a healthier lifestyle. You may be required to participate in long-term follow-up plans that include monitoring your nutrition, your lifestyle and behavior, and your medical conditions. Ultimately remember that surgery is not the answer to all of your weight issues, it's merely an aid or a beginning, YOU, my friend, have to put an end to your issues.

And keep in mind that bariatric surgery is expensive. Check with your health insurance plan or your regional Medicare or Medicaid office to find out if your policy covers such surgery.

Risks: As with any major surgery, all weight-loss surgeries pose potential health risks, both in the short term and long term.

Risks associated with the procedures can include:

•Excessive bleeding

•Infection

•Adverse reactions to anesthesia

•Blood clots

•Lung or breathing problems

•Leaks in your gastrointestinal system

•Death (rare)

Personally I have had none of these.

Longer term risks and complications of weight-loss surgery vary depending on the type of surgery. They can include:

•*Bowel obstruction*

•*Dumping syndrome, (causing diarrhea, nausea or vomiting)*

•*Gallstones*

•*Hernias*

•*Low blood sugar (hypoglycemia)*

•Malnutrition

•Stomach perforation

•Ulcers

•Vomiting

•Death (rare)

Now I would not be honest if I left you thinking all was perfect with me. The items in italics listed above are what I did have. Why? Because I felt so good that I left the instructions of my doctor and nutritionist behind and went on to discover my own America! I tried foods too early. I discovered what I really could no longer and should no longer eat. And I also discovered that although I was getting thin and beautiful in my own eyes, eating was a necessary requirement for life! Malnutrition results in death, a state where I didn't want to go! We will go into some of the things on the list a little later.

Gastric bypass and other types of weight-loss surgery are done in the hospital, not a clinic or on a kitchen table! I have to say that because so many people are monumentally desperate that they will take the word of anyone who says they will make them thin and beautiful by giving them weight loss surgery cheap! You get what you pay for. IT'S DONE IN A HOSPITAL!!!

There are actually three popular types of weight loss surgeries. Each surgical procedure have their own benefits and risks. Here is a comparison for you to review. Use this general information and by all means talk with your doctor to help decide if, and which, surgery option is appropriate for you.

Bariatric Surgical Procedure Similarities

SKINNY WOMEN ARE NOT CREATED EQUAL

The following information is an overview of the differences between surgical weight loss options. You should discuss with your doctor the benefits as well as the risks of weight loss surgery and decide what's right for you.

The specifics of your surgery depend on your individual situation, the type of weight-loss surgery you have, and the hospital's or doctor's practices. Some weight-loss surgeries are done with traditional large, or open, incisions in your abdomen. Today, most types of bariatric surgery are performed laparoscopically. A laparoscope is a small, tubular instrument with a camera attached. The laparoscope is inserted through small incisions in the abdomen. The tiny camera on the tip of the laparoscope allows the surgeon to see and operate inside your abdomen without making the traditional large incisions. Laparoscopic surgery can make your recovery faster and shorter, but it's not suitable for everyone.

Surgery usually takes several hours. After surgery, you awaken in a recovery room, where medical staff monitors you for any complications. Your hospital stay may last from three to five days. Still, all forms of weight-loss surgery are major procedures that can pose serious risks and side effects. Again, you must make permanent healthy changes to your diet and get regular exercise to help ensure the long-term success of bariatric surgery.

(For a visual of each of the surgeries, you can go online. I encourage you to please do your own research before making this life changing decision.)

1.   **<u>Gastric Bypass</u>**: In this procedure, the surgeon creates a small stomach pouch and attaches a section of the small intestine directly to the pouch.

This allows food to bypass a portion of the small intestine.

How it works in helping you to lose weight is by creating a smaller stomach pouch. The gastric bypass limits the amount of food that can be eaten at one time, so you feel full sooner and stay full longer. By bypassing a portion of the small intestine, your body also absorbs fewer calories. As you eat less, your body will stop storing excess calories and start using its fat supply for energy.

How it affects digestion is by reducing the amount of calories, in the form of nutrients, which are being absorbed.

2.   **Gastric Sleeve**: During the sleeve procedure, a thin vertical sleeve of stomach is created using a stapling device. The sleeve is about the size of a banana, and the rest of the stomach is removed.

How it works to help you lose weight is by creating a smaller stomach pouch. The sleeve gastrectomy procedure limits the amount of food that can be eaten at one time, so you feel full sooner and stay full longer. As you eat less food, your body will stop storing excess calories and start using its fat supply for energy.

How it affects digestion is not much at all. It does not significantly affect normal digestion and absorption. Food passes through the digestive tract in the usual order, allowing it to be fully absorbed in the body.

3.   **Gastric Lap Band**: The gastric band wraps around the upper part of the stomach, dividing the stomach into a small upper pouch that holds about ½ cup of food and a larger lower stomach. The degree of band tightness affects how much food you can eat and

the length of time it takes for food to leave the stomach pouch.

How it works to help you lose weight is by creating a smaller stomach pouch. The band limits the amount of food that can be eaten at one time, so you feel full sooner and stay full longer. As you eat less food, your body will stop storing excess calories and start using its fat energy supply.

How it affects digestion is not significant. I does not affect normal digestion and absorption. Food passes through the digestive tract in the usual order, allowing it to be fully absorbed in the body.

General anesthesia is used for all weight-loss surgery. This means you're unconscious during the procedure IN THE HOSPITAL!

After surgery, you generally won't be allowed to eat for one to two days so that your stomach and digestive system can heal. Then, you'll follow a specific diet for about 12 weeks...that's TWELVE WEEKS!! The diet begins with liquids only, then progresses to ground-up or soft foods, and finally to regular foods. You may have many restrictions or limits on how much and what you can eat and drink.

You'll also have frequent medical checkups to monitor your health in the first several months after surgery. You may need laboratory testing, blood work and various exams.

You may experience changes as your body reacts to the rapid weight loss in the first three to six months after gastric bypass or other weight-loss surgery, including:

•Body aches

•Feeling tired, as if you have the flu

•Feeling cold

•Dry skin

•Hair thinning and hair loss

•Mood changes

Bariatric surgeries can provide long-term weight loss **if you cooperate and allow the surgery to do what it was intended.** The amount of weight you lose depends on your type of surgery and your change in lifestyle habits. It may be possible to lose half, or even more, of your excess weight within two years.

In addition to weight loss, gastric bypass surgery may improve or resolve conditions often related to, not only obesity but being in poor health from the start.

Many Doctors have noted the significant changes in blood pressure in their patients within the first ten days after surgery. And gastric bypass surgery can also improve your ability to perform routine daily activities, which could help improve your quality of life.

When weight-loss surgery doesn't work, what do you do?

Gastric bypass and other weight-loss surgeries don't always work as well as you might have hoped. For one thing, although rare, something during or after the procedure may go wrong. For instance, the adjustable band may fail to work properly. If a weight-loss procedure doesn't work right or stops working, you may not lose weight and you may develop serious health problems. Keep all of your scheduled follow-up appointments after weight-loss surgery. If you notice that you aren't losing weight or you develop complications, see your doctor immediately. Your weight loss can be monitored and factors potentially contributing to your lack of weight loss evaluated.

It's also possible to not lose enough weight or to regain weight after any type of weight-loss surgery, even if the procedure itself works correctly. This weight gain can happen **if you don't follow the recommended lifestyle changes.** To help avoid regaining weight, you must make permanent healthy changes in your diet and get regular physical activity and exercise. If you frequently snack on high-calorie foods, for instance, you may have inadequate weight loss. Be honest with yourself! Make the change and keep the change!   ***

<u>WHAT GOES IN SHOULD NOT COME OUT</u>

We...us folks as a nation of people are part of **S.A.D.:** *THE STANDARD AMERICAN DIET!* And it goes something like this: We eat the Standard American Diet every day and are surprised when we don't feel well. We then go to the Standard American Doctor who gives us the upsetting news about our newly revealed Standard American Disease. So then this doctor, prescribes for us the Standard American Drug which has awful side effects and slowly causes us to die the Standard American Death! This is SAD!! True enough we may have inherited a family condition which might be the gun, but poor eating habits definitely pulls the trigger!

After surgery it is imperative that you immediately begin to cooperate with the diet plan that is set before you. How you start your race, many time will be how you end your race, right back at the beginning. It is never too late to start, however, the later you start, the longer you will take to get to your finish line. **<u>Just get started.</u>**

I had a friend who had the surgery and on the way home, her son had B-B-Q ribs with extra sauce waiting for her in the car, by her request! She wanted to "simply chew the meat from each bone, suck off the sauce and spit it all out!" She declared it was simple and innocent. She just wanted the flavor! This is on the way home following surgery! And she had all of the discomfort that came with it. She didn't care, she wanted what she wanted. Today she is bigger than before surgery. She never got a chance to start her race.

You must cooperate with your surgery and the diet to follow. Not only that, but there are nutrients that you will not be able to absorb from your foods because you can't get enough food in your system. So along with your diet, you must take supplements. Not to cooperate with this will leave you weak, irritable, feeling lousy, not being able to thrive and ultimately live the life you are trying to carve out for yourself because you don't have the energy to do so.

The list of vitamins and supplements are as follows, at least this is the list that I was given and the list that I worked from that aided in my weight loss success:

YOU MUST HAVE THEM FOR YOUR NUTRITIONAL NEEDS. TO NEGLECT THEM MEANS TO NEGLECT YOUR HEALTH. Whether you have surgery or not you need vitamins and supplements because the foods we eat today lack the nutrition needed for our bodies to be at their optimum best.

Vitamins

- Multi-vitamin

- B12-1000mg

- B1 Thiamine (Super B complex 100mg)

SKINNY WOMEN ARE NOT CREATED EQUAL

- Vitamin D-2000 IU

- Calcium Citrate 1200-500mg

- Biotin-1000 mcg

- Folic Acid

- Iron

- Omega 3, 6, 9

It doesn't matter where you get them from, however, DO NOT PURCHASE THEM FROM THE CORNER DRUG STORE. It would be far better for you to purchase them from a whole-food/health food store or a wholefood/health food distributor. Most of the time, these drug store or even big-box store vitamins, although convenient, may be synthetic or man-made and are not as advantageous to your body as vitamins and supplements that are 100% natural or organic. The reason this is important is in order for the supplements to benefit you, they must be **bioavailable**, which means that they are 100% beneficial to your body. If you take vitamins in and you see them again when you eliminate, your body did not absorb them at all.

<u>Weight Loss Surgery Diet</u>: What to eat after the surgery?

The gastric bypass diet is designed for people who are recovering from gastric bypass surgery to help them heal but eating habits MUST change. Your doctor or a registered dietitian can help you with a gastric bypass diet by guiding your meal planning.

A gastric bypass diet specifies what type and how much food you can eat at each meal. Closely following your gastric bypass diet can help you lose weight safely.

<u>**Purpose:**</u>

The gastric bypass diet has several purposes:

•To allow the staple line in your stomach to heal without being stretched by the food you eat

•To get you accustomed to eating the smaller amounts of food that can be digested comfortably and safely in your smaller stomach

•To help you lose weight and avoid gaining excess weight

•To avoid side effects and complications

<u>**Diet Details:**</u>

Most commonly, the gastric bypass diet has four phases to help you ease back into eating solid foods. How quickly you move from one step to the next depends on how fast your body heals and adjusts to the change in eating patterns. You can usually start eating regular foods with a firmer texture about three months after surgery.

After gastric bypass or other weight-loss surgery, you must pay extra attention to signs that you feel hungry or full. You may develop some food intolerances or aversions.

Phase 1: Liquid diet

You won't be allowed to eat for one to two days after gastric bypass surgery so that your stomach can start to heal. After that, while you're still in the hospital, you start a diet of liquids and semisolid foods to see how you tolerate foods after surgery.

SKINNY WOMEN ARE NOT CREATED EQUAL

Foods you may be able to have on phase 1 of the gastric bypass diet include:

•Broth

•Unsweetened juice

•Milk

Popsicles

•Strained cream soup

•Sugar-free gelatin

During phase 1, (two to four weeks), sip fluids slowly and drink only 2 to 3 ounces, (59 to 89 milliliters, or mL) at a time. Don't drink carbonated or caffeinated beverages. And don't eat and drink at the same time. Wait about 30 minutes after a meal to drink anything.

Initially I was not hungry at all. I didn't even want water but I had to force myself to sip that several times a day for the first few days. Eventually I moved onto the other liquids and was on them for about 2 weeks.

Dr. Jerry told me that it would be ok for my stomach not to have food in it for a few days. My body would be eating on its own fat for that length of time. Quite naturally I could understand that, I had so much of it!

I once met a man who had the same surgery that I had but was given the wrong instructions. After his second week, he was told that he could go back to his former diet. He wanted to discuss why he felt so bad all the time. I asked what he had eaten the night before. He said, "Just meatloaf"! ***Just meatloaf!? After 2 weeks!?*** He probably went to that "Bad Doctor"!

Along with sipping the liquids, I would get out of bed and take a few steps down the hall each day. I wouldn't tackle the stairs but I could walk up and down the hall from bedroom to bedroom in my home without much help if I took my time.

I had 6 tiny incisions in my stomach cavity. I wasn't in much pain from those, I was in discomfort from the stitches inside and I was weak because I didn't have food or fuel in my system.

What I found to be very interesting was I was hungry at breakfast only because **it was breakfast time**, not because I was actually hungry. And then at about 11:30, my brain said that it was lunch time and that I should be hungry, but I wasn't. And of course at dinner time, my eyes glanced at my watch so that I could confirm that it was time for me to eat dinner, again not that I was hungry for it but it was time for it. We are programmed that way all throughout our lives. From Kindergarten through our adult work experience, we look at the time and know it's food time regardless of if we are really hungry or not!

Phase 2: Pureed foods

Once you're able to tolerate liquid foods for a few days, you can begin to eat pureed (mashed up) foods. During this two- to four-week-long phase, you can only eat foods that have the consistency of a smooth paste or a thick liquid, without any solid pieces of food in the mixture.

To puree your foods, choose solid foods that will blend well, such as:

•Lean ground meats

•Beans

•Fish

•Egg whites

•Yogurt

•Soft fruits and vegetables

•Cottage cheese

Blend the solid food with a liquid, such as:

•Water

•Fat-free milk

•Juice with no sugar added

•Broth

•Fat-free gravy

Keep in mind that your digestive system might still be sensitive to spicy foods or dairy products. If you'd like to eat these foods during this phase, add them into your diet slowly and in small amounts.

Phase 3: Soft, solid foods

With your doctor's permission, after a few weeks of pureed foods, you can add soft, solid foods to your diet. If you can mash your food with a fork, it's soft enough to include in this phase of your diet.

During this phase, your diet can include:

•Ground or finely diced meats

•Canned or soft, fresh fruit

•Cooked vegetables

You usually eat soft foods for eight weeks before eating foods of regular consistency with firmer texture, as recommended by your dietitian or doctor.

Phase 4: Solid foods

After about eight weeks on the gastric bypass diet, you can gradually return to eating firmer foods. You may find that you still have difficulty eating spicier foods or foods with crunchy textures. Start slowly with regular foods to see what foods you can tolerate.

Avoid these foods. Even at this stage after surgery, avoid these foods:

•Nuts and seeds

•Popcorn

•Dried fruits

•Sodas and carbonated beverages

•Granola

•Stringy or fibrous vegetables, such as celery, broccoli, corn or cabbage

•Tough meats or meats with gristle

•Breads

These foods are discouraged because they typically aren't well tolerated in the weeks after surgery and might cause gastrointestinal symptoms. Over time, you may be able to try some of these foods again, with the guidance of your doctor.

A return to normal

Three to four months after weight-loss surgery, you may be able to start returning to a normal healthy diet, depending on your situation and any foods you may not be able to tolerate. It's possible that foods that initially irritated your stomach after surgery may become more tolerable as your stomach continues to heal.

Throughout the phases.

To ensure that you get enough vitamins and minerals and keep your weight-loss goals on track, at each phase of the gastric bypass diet, you should:

•**Keep meals small.** Each meal should include about a third to a half-cup of food. Make sure you eat only the recommended amounts and stop eating before you feel full.

•**Take recommended vitamin and mineral supplements.** Because a portion of your small intestine is bypassed after surgery, your body won't be able to absorb enough nutrients from your food. You'll need to take a multivitamin supplement every day for the rest of your life, so talk to your doctor about what type of multivitamin might be right for you, and whether you might need to take additional supplements, such as calcium. The supplements that I use are whole-food products and have worked so well for me that I decided to sell them on a large scale. And they are not just for post-surgery patients, they are beneficial for overall better health, weight-loss for those who have gained their weight back and weight maintenance. They have caused my hair, skin and nails to become stronger, my skin then becomes softer and my overall health to stabilize.

•**Drink liquids between meals.** Drinking liquids with your meals can cause pain, nausea and vomiting as well as dumping syndrome. Also, drinking too much liquid at or around mealtime can leave you feeling overly full and prevent you from eating enough. Expect to drink at least 6 to 8 cups (48 to 64 ounces or 1.4 to 1.9 liters) of fluids a day to prevent dehydration.

•Eat and drink slowly. Eating or drinking too quickly may cause the dumping syndrome — when foods and liquids enter your small intestine rapidly and in larger amounts than normal, causing nausea, vomiting, dizziness, sweating and eventually diarrhea. To prevent dumping syndrome, choose foods and liquids low in fat and sugar, (Preferably fat and sugar free), eat and drink slowly, and wait 30 to 45 minutes before or after each meal to drink liquids. Take at least 30 minutes to eat your meals and 30 to 60 minutes to drink 1 cup (237 milliliters) of liquid. Avoid foods high in fat and sugar, such as non-diet soda, candy, candy bars and ice cream.

My husband and I were invited to a couple's dinner a few weeks following surgery. There was a "sweets" table, of which I knew I could not partake, but there was a buffet of meats. Among those meats was a dish of BBQ wings. Harmless!

I got my saucer and got 3 or 4 of the smallest wings I could find. OOOH holy cow were they good. After about 10 minutes, I asked my husband if the heat was turned up. I began to sweat and had this strange feeling in the top of my stomach. I excused myself and promptly went to the restroom. As soon as I lifted the lid and opened my mouth, all of the chicken and sauce can rolling out. I mean rolling out without effort. When I was finished, I could taste all of the sugar in that sauce. That was my first experience with the "dumping syndrome", a great mechanism if you ask me. When you shouldn't have eaten something, sweat, discomfort and then out it comes...usually.

•Chew food thoroughly. The new opening that leads from your stomach into your intestine is very small, and larger pieces of food can block the opening. Blockages prevent food from leaving your stomach and can cause vomiting, nausea and abdominal pain.

Take small bites of food and chew them to a pureed consistency before swallowing. If you can't chew the food thoroughly, don't swallow it.

•Try new foods one at a time. After surgery, certain foods may cause nausea, pain and vomiting or may block the opening of the stomach. The ability to tolerate foods varies from person to person. Try one new food at a time and chew thoroughly before swallowing. If a food causes discomfort, don't eat it.

•Focus on high-protein foods. Immediately after your surgery, eating high-protein foods can help heal your wounds, regrow muscle and skin, and prevent hair loss. High-protein, low-fat choices remain a good long-term diet option after your surgery, as well. Try adding lean cuts of beef, chicken, pork, fish or beans to your diet. Low-fat cheese, cottage cheese and yogurts also are good protein sources. Every meal that I eat is made up of Protein, *Protein*, **Protein** first, then vegetable and then whatever else if available. If I happen to order a pizza, I have made myself fall in love with vegetable, thin crust. 2 to 4 slices is all I can get in and that's all I can do, even after 10 years since having surgery. And my choice of beverages are either lemon water or an unsweetened tea mixed with a little lemonade which restaurants call an Arnold Palmer.

•Avoid breaded foods. After your surgery, it may be difficult for your digestive system to tolerate foods that are high in fat and heavily breaded. Fried foods are very hard to digest, especially with unknown oil. Over time, fried anything is where most people begin to gain their weight back. They build up a tolerance for the breading and the oil.

A few years back, my mom had a mild stroke. Between myself and my younger sister, I was the logical one to take care of her during the day. Her favorite food was fried chicken wings and a Pepsi. With me feeling so emotional about her condition, I couldn't say, "No", to her food requests. Unfortunately when she ate fried chicken, I ate fried chicken...3 to 4 days a week. I started out at 125lbs. 2 years later she was back to good health but I was 198lbs and depressed. 73lbs of fried chicken in 2 years after putting in so much work and dedication would make anyone depressed. ***

LURCH AND THE CREEPY NUN

So came the day of surgery. I was so "geeked" and nervous but never afraid. I had done my research and I had my husband's support as well as my Pastor's prayers. I had full confidence in Dr. Jerry and his team and above all I knew God was with me.

If you think you have no one to support you, highlight these paragraphs: A.) First and foremost, make sure you have done your research. You can't even consider a matter if you don't know all of the facts. You have to know exactly what you are getting in to. B.) Then, you must know who your doctor is and have full confidence in that team of people. If you have not met your doctor, but have only spoken or met with the nurse or the assistant team, **STOP!** Cancel your appointment and demand a sit-down with your doctor. There is no such thing as he is too busy to meet with you. If he is always in surgery and cannot meet with you, he is just making money and not relationships. He cares nothing for his patients. Hint! Hint! Clue! Clue!

And, C.) The other thing you must have if you have no other physical support person is absolutely know that *you have GOD with you.* He is going into surgery with you and He will bring you out of surgery. You must have a good frame of mind going in. If you go in with death or dying on your mind, your outcome might not as you expect. Your mental disposition during surgery will continue to rehearse itself while you are under anesthesia and bring you out on the wrong side of confidence. Depression will set in and you will have set yourself up for failure even before you have begun your journey.

I had a weight loss student, Susan, who desperately wanted to lose weight. I taught a 6 week weight-loss class and I became very fond of her. She had no family or close friends to support her. During that time, I promised her that I would be with her when she went into surgery and when she came out of surgery. I was absolutely definite on that promise.

She was very frightened of the whole ordeal and occasionally leaned on me for support. In her current state she didn't want to be a burden on anyone. She was confined to a motorized wheel chair because of her weight and needed help getting around. Her heart's desire was to be part of a loving family someday.

It was around the first of January and the day came for her surgery. And wouldn't you know it, I could not get there at all because of a Polar Vortex Storm that blew through Chicago and closed down many of the streets, schools and businesses. I was absolutely sick that I could not be there. My husband told me not to make a move towards that hospital which was downtown, but to stay home.

I felt absolutely awful that Susan had to go in and come out of surgery alone. But what I realized was that she was never alone. God was with her completely. I spent the next few days kicking myself for not being there when I gave my word but it absolutely just could not be helped. Didn't God know that a Polar Vortex was going to blow through Chicago? Heck He blew it through there in the first place! Didn't he know that I had given my word and that she'd be all alone? What I've come to understand in that type of situation is that for her journey, this is her journey. If I had gone, my heart would have gotten wrapped up in her journey and I would have been so moved with compassion that I would have done the next thing and the next thing for her. I would have also not allowed her to support herself, stand on her own 2 feet, toughen her own skin, strengthen her own backbone, and gain some new wits about how to maneuver in this new life on her own. In short, I would have been her new crutch. This was a journey that she had to take. The storm with whipped up just for that purpose.

I know what to do and what not to do and I probably would not have allowed her to do much of anything for herself. I would not have allowed her to fall or make any mistakes. I would not have allowed the baby to walk because I would have cared for the baby just that much. Sometimes it's for you to jump in, but sometimes as much as you want to jump in, and my heart wanted to badly be there for her, but because I was "all in", God pulled me "all out"! I certainly keep in touch via text and she probably felt neglected and unsupported. But it was all for her purpose, just as in the case of caring for my mother. Things unfolded in such a way that I was absolutely pulled out. Life happens beyond our control sometimes and if I had not been pulled out, I would have gained my weight and more back. Both Mom and Susan needed to figure out some things on their own.

So what is my point? My point is that although you may feel that you don't have the support that you need. Sometimes, you are your support for the reasons that God is orchestrating. You may not see that in the beginning, but on the other side is peace and amazement! And because it's solely your journey, it is doing great things to strengthen you mentally, emotionally and physically that you didn't know were there. Don't fight it, just go with it.

You don't want to be around people who don't support you or those who would seek to sabotage you especially the days heading into surgery. I heard of a man who opted for a huge steak and potato two days before his surgery. Bad idea! If you must have that "last big meal", celebrate a week before because you have to clean out your colon. The surgeons don't want to go in and have a mess on their hands...literally!

So my instructions were to go to Walgreens and pick up Magnesium Citrate Saline Laxative Oral Solution in Lemon flavor. I had to purchase 2 bottles and drink both of them. Simple right? Yuck to the Max!!!! To get them down I had to dilute them in water and pour them over ice. Let me warn you, when they begin to work, stay close to the bathroom.... ***YOU WILL EXPLODE and MANY TIMES!!!!!*** My meals consisted of broth and water...just for 2 days. I could do that.

Day of surgery came. I was so nervous. My life Is getting ready to change FOREVER!!!! People are going to see me different FOREVER!!! At the time I didn't know that this was just an aid. I sincerely thought this was an answer and in the deep, deep recesses of my mind, I thought this would MAKE ME SKINNY PERMANENTLY AND FOREVER!!!!

Once in my hospital gown, I was wheeled into a "holding room". Each of the team members that would be contributing to my surgery came in and spoke with me to reassure me that all would be well. They were comforting and encouraging. My husband, Mike was right there holding my hand.

And then it happened. This creepy nun came in and begin praying for me as if I had died on the table. Her responsibility was to pray that my spirit would go to heaven. But what about my mental state right now? She had all but pronounced me gone!!! I had to stop her mid-stream and tell her I was all good. My Pastor had already prayed for me and I didn't need her to pray for me. I absolutely did not want that on my mind going into surgery.

As if that wasn't enough, then a Priest... Lurch from the Adam's Family, came in where she had left off. And again he began to give me my last rights. I put my hand up and stopped him. My husband even told him we were all good. We thanked him but told him, "No Thanks."

You have to have your mind right when you go in so that you can settle your spirit during the surgery and come out on top. Even if there are medical issues during surgery, your spirit is well and can work "with God" instead of against God. You need all the support you can get...even self-support.

If you are afraid, say that. Tell someone that you are afraid. Go to a close friend, a Pastor, your doctor, someone and get that fear out. To avoid it only allows it to mount and bubble over at the wrong time. Have you ever seen a person have a panic attack out of nowhere after a major event when they seemed cool and calm? Just like the Florida Evans character in Good Times, the 70's sitcom. When James, her husband died, she didn't deal with her grief and anger right off because it was too much. She had to be strong for her family. But when it was all over days later, she had a glass bowl in her hands, she smashed it and screamed, "DAMN! DAMN! DAMN!" Too often we have tried to be strong for everyone else and show no fear or weakness when what we need to do is rely on the people around us for support and help us get through it. Don't lie to yourself, tell someone what you need.

Remember this is the beginning of the new you. You are no longer being the unnecessary super-woman supporting everyone else and not allowing anyone to support you. TELL SOMEONE WHAT YOU NEED!

When I came out of surgery, everything was foggy. I remember Mike taking the surgical tape, which held my oxygen tube, off of my face. I remember saying, "pain", but I don't remember feeling pain.

The nursing team moved me from the gurney to the bed and did all the medical I-V things necessary to keep me comfortable. And then after a couple of hours, I woke up. I remember being extremely excited!! See, if my mental state was jacked up and not right going in, I would not have been right coming out.

As I was waking up, the nurse was coming in and asking me to sit up! NO! NO! I couldn't do it. Now I could feel the pain!!!! The nurse gave me the choice to sit and recover in a recliner instead of the bed. Whoo!... that was so much better! Along with sitting in the chair, I had to wear these electric boots that would massage my legs to make sure I had no blood clots set into my veins.

I was in the hospital for about 3 days and had no desire to eat what so ever. Dr. Jerry had me drink this liquid and stand in front of a machine that could view the liquid going through my new system to make sure there were no leaks. And they gave me blood thinning shots to keep me from having blood clots. And I would continue to give them to myself at home for at least a month to make sure I didn't develop clots later. ***

SAILING GOOD

During surgery the team placed a tube in my stomach cavity to drain any fluid and it emptied into a little plastic bulb that was taped to the largest incision on my left side. When I left the hospital, I was given instructions on how to care for the incisions, and how to give myself the daily blood thinner shots.

About 10 days to 2 weeks after being released, I went back to Dr. Jerry for my follow up. There were other women in the waiting room all bent over with pain and various degrees of not feeling well. I was feeling terrific! I came bouncing in, happy and ready to detach from that little bulb and get on with moving into the world of the skinny me!!!

Dr. Jerry asked me, "What the heck are you on?" I just told him that I was feeling great and I was on my liquid supplements, not eating anything but just sipping liquids and my supplements. He told me to keep it up!

After my exam and he removed the bulb and the tube, I left his office to go on to discover my own America, my own world of freedom from the world of fat! I had no thought that this was not going to work or that I would be challenged somehow on any food level. I thought it was conquered through surgery. So Onward I charged. I sailed away into the wild blue yonder in my speed boat to "Thin-hood Island".

Over the next year I went down to 125lbs. and each day of that year was a tremendous wow! I'd go to bed and wake up having lost another 2 or 3 lbs. The world of thin is so different when you enter in as an adult then if you grew up in it.

When you grow up thin you just move through life sitting where you want, entering and exiting when you want. Pulling clothes off the rack, knowing they should fit but you'll try them on just to be sure. And the best yet, crossing your legs to think, to be more comfortable or just to be cute!

A heavy person has to prepare their mind every day for the simplest tasks that the skinny world takes for granted. What's bad is that the heavy person doesn't even know that they are doing it. It's a survival routine that they have unconsciously mastered and until you have gone from fat to skinny will you see the full scope of this mastery.

As I mentioned in an earlier chapter, I learned how to maneuver around in the world without hitting someone in the head with my hip as I passed by. What's sad is far too many people either have not mastered it, have given up mastering it or there simply isn't enough room in many situations to avoid the application. Once again, the world isn't set up for the obese even though 70% of the world is larger than life.

I remember being in Worship Service at my church as I was losing weight and I had on a wonderful powder blue fitted dress that was an awesome size 8. I was still adjusting to my bra size and my undergarments so I had not gotten them quite right. But all-in-all I thought I looked fantastic. Going from a 28W to a 8P in a year was amazing not just to me but to every single person around me.

I was smack-dab in the front and bouncing and clapping away to the music and I just happened to look down and my "old girls" had slipped down below the bra line! I don't know how long I had been that way but I was surely a sight in that fitted light blue dress! It was all I could do to cross my arms over myself and make it through the crowd of fellow parishioners and to the bathroom so that I could pull everything back into place, tie a knot, pin it up or pin it down so that I could get back to my place in Praise and Worship!

I didn't go out and buy a ton of clothes after a few pounds were gone because I didn't know where I was going to end up. I didn't know if 125lbs was it or if I was going to lose more or gain some back. I just didn't know and Dr. Jerry couldn't tell me that either. He said time would tell me that. He said I would decide if I'm too skinny at 125lbs. or if I want to lose another 5lbs.

I remember one day going into a K-Mart story to see just what size jeans I could wear after having lost some 45lbs. I didn't know where to begin so I pulled off the shelf a 22, 20, 18 and 16 W's. ALL OF THEM WERE TOO BIG!!! I began crying and dancing in the dressing room right then and there. As I was losing weight I had been tacking up my skirts and sweatpants until they became just too ridiculous. So officially Mr. K-Mart said that I was a size 14 and not in the "Women" ..."14 Misses" and I was insanely excited!

I only bought a few things that I called "my staples" that I could mix and match as I went down in size. Otherwise it would have seriously been a waste of money. ***

<u>AM I MENTAL?</u>

I was given the opportunity to speak at a Support Group for Weight Loss Surgery some weeks ago. My talk was on "There Is More to Your Story than What They See". It's more than keeping those burger and fries away. There is a mental side that many weight loss professionals don't really address, especially if they have not had the surgery themselves.

Story: There was this dog who came running into the house with this rabbit. Both he and the rabbit were muddy. It was obvious that the dog had been playing with it and killed it.

The guy who owned the dog knew the rabbit belonged to the next door neighbor so he managed to get the rabbit from the dog and wash it, dry it and was able to put it back into the rabbit cage before the owners got home from work.

Later that evening, the neighbor who owned the rabbit screamed out and ran with the rabbit in her hand to the guys' back door. He opened the door and pretended not to know what was going on. He said, "What's the trouble?" She said, "Look, our rabbit, our rabbit! It died last week. We buried it in the yard and somehow it managed to get back into the cage!"

There is more to your story than what people think they see. People don't know what has happened to you to bring you to where you are right now. No one knows what's going on inside you as you deal with or work through your weight or health journey. The transformation is monumental and people and perhaps even you think that *you should be able to just walk right out of your fat clothes and fat thoughts and into a new set of skinny threads and be free, mind, body and soul! It's not going to happen like that.*

The #1 question that I was asked after my lecture was how did I mentally deal with my body changing when it came to the outside world? Not to sound vain but I never thought I was unattractive, even at nearly 300lbs. But honey, when I got that weight off, you couldn't tell me I wasn't eye-candy, even to myself!

I was in a unique place with that because I already had a husband that loved me fat or skinny. My adjustment came from the attention I got beyond my husband. And I'd be lying to you if I told you that I didn't get much attention on the streets but it didn't rattle me because I was already getting attention at home.

So with that let me tell you, if your mind isn't on straight or you are not getting it at home, you will lose your mind when you lose your weight! The attention will blow you away...but don't let it because it will take you up to let you down. If I didn't say it before, let me say it now, DON'T BELIEVE THE HYPE!!!

The attention you didn't get before will be overwhelming to you now. You will want to believe all the words of every Gorgeous George out there. But let me tell you he is just a "Gimp"! He is accustomed to beautiful women falling for him and his smooth beautiful words. However, you are not accustomed to beautiful men falling for you!! There is a verse of scripture that says, *"Beloved, believe not every spirit, but try the spirits whether they are of God:"*   1 John 4:1

If they were your friends before and have remained as such, then you are all good but if they paid you not the time of day before and now they seem to fall at your feet, they are shallow. Also, if you have just met them since losing weight, don't be too quick to believe their words of admiration or dedication to you. They don't know you and you don't know them.

You are at a vulnerable stage, understand that and accept that. Own it and be okay with it. If you let anyone take advantage of you because of it, whether male or female, you will fall into a hole of depression and jeopardize all the weight you have lost and all the self-esteem you have gained. You will have allowed hurts to come in and will have opened doors that you didn't know were there. And now you sincerely need someone to take you by the hand to help you walk back out. You, my darling might have to do it on your own. Not that you can't but because of your own desperation and a need not to be lonely, this will be the hardest mental work of your life!

It is already grueling because you are changing and reinventing anyway but to add to that self-destruction, ignorance or desperation and loneliness makes recovery and rediscovery of self so much longer and harder. But perhaps that's the road YOU have to take anyway.

Surgery, weight loss, healing and recovery is going on in more than just the lower part of your body, it's going on in your head too! ***

<u>*LIFE HAPPENS*</u>

I'm going along with my weight loss and having a ball. I'm down to a 6/8 petite! Holy Cow! Then life happens! My beautiful mom had a stroke. I found myself in the position to have to care for not only my 77 year old mom, but her severely handicapped 73 year old brother, my uncle and my 15 year old handicapped brother as well.

While I was not strong enough to do so, I couldn't just leave them to be cared for by the State. At the time I just jumped right in and cared for them. Certainly my sister did what she could and my husband was there to support me and was a tremendous help when he was not at work but I carried the burden of her care 24/7 if not physically definitely mentally.

Mom had her complete wits about her and she was adamant that she was not going to a home of any kind. They all were going to stay together and in her home with her. So...I nursed them all 12 hours a day 6 ½ days a week!

This went on for 2 years. She got stronger and enjoyed the security of me being there but the flip side of it was....I began to gain weight. Why? Because I had to shut down all that I had been doing for me to care for them. I sat by their side for 12 hours every day. I cooked and cleaned and did what a home care person does for handicapped elderly people.

Depression set in like never before and I didn't like it. She couldn't help her stroke and my uncle and brother couldn't help their conditions but nonetheless, I was in the worse mental state of my life. I actually began taking more medication than my mom. Medication to get up in the morning, medication for the pain in my back. Medication for stress and medication to put me to sleep at night. It was terrible. And to make matters worse, I ate and I ate.

When it was all said and done I had gained back 70lbs. I was so disappointed in myself and had nowhere to go emotionally to get an understanding of what to do to get my mental straight. At the same time I couldn't leave my mom but I had to do something.

I had abandoned all vitamins, supplements and right eating habits and had replaced them with my brother's junk food, my mother's binge eating and I had even gone back to fast-food eating after I had left for the night. Depression is a monster and a rope that ties you down or binds you up.

On my one day off a week all I'd do was lay in the bed, with my dog and watch television while my family lived life without me. It was awful and I was getting fatter, sicker and my family was getting more and more resentful. Something had to give.

Out of the blue one day, I was standing in the kitchen and mom went totally nuts on me and told me to leave her house! She was sick of me taking control of her affairs, controlling her house and she wanted me gone. So I packed up my few things and I left. When I tell you I was devastated. I sniveled and wailed the 45 minute drive home.

I called my Pastor and she told me that many times the oldest child in the family takes on more than they should even to their own detriment. I wouldn't leave so God had to literally kick me out. It was getting dangerous for my health and they were getting too dependent on me and they need more care than I could ever give.

I cried for a few days, got through it and set a brand new plan for myself. The first thing I did was began walking 20 minutes a day for about 3 days a week. Nothing on the weekends. I did this for about 3 months just to get my mind and body back in line. I knew that if I jumped back in too quickly after sitting for 2 years I'll be overwhelmed and quit.

Then I was given a Cleanse Tea to rid my body of the toxins and junk that I had been eating. Not only was I depressed for 2 years, I hit a "Fat Patch"! Finally I lined up my vitamins and supplements and put myself on a plan of consistency. All in all it took me about 8 months to a year to get that fat patch of 70lbs off.

Mom and I are great now. She has help coming in for the three of them. But it would have never happened had I stayed. If I had stayed, I probably would be the one needing State aide!

Life is going to hit so expect it. Your weight lose plans might get detoured, altered, hit a snag, a roadblock or even a brick wall. Take a moment, compose yourself, regroup and either start over or reset your sail and continue on. You will be ok...... **JUST DON'T QUIT!!!!!** If you quit, you will never get there.   ***

<u>*SUPPLEMENTS*</u>

In the last chapter I talked about using a cleanse tea to rid my body of toxins before I began my weight loss for the second time. See the first time, Dr. Jerry had me clean my colon for medical reasons, this time, and every time I feel the need it's gentler, healthier and more fulfilling.

When I attacked my weight loss this last time, I had a different mindset. The first time, I was filled with desperation and put my weight loss in the hands of Dr. Jerry. This time my weight loss was solely in my own hands.

I have heard of people having the surgery **multiple times** and that's just ludicrous! If you don't get it right the first time, back up and start over, but not with surgery; with a new plan of action. God himself created the world and when he saw that folks went nuts, he wiped them out and started over. He didn't cancel out the earth, he just started over with new people. Get a new plan and start over. Not new surgery, *just a new plan.*

When you have had weight loss surgery, or even attempt to just lose weight period, you must take your vitamins and supplements. I listed them in an earlier chapter. And when you get out of whack with your weight, and you will, begin again more intelligently. I was looking for things to help me stay on track with my health. I didn't want to fall off ever again. I found a supplement that would do just that. It had all the vitamins necessary for those who have had the surgery plus a few extra things.

Whatever supplements you settle on, make sure it's right for you and that it will include what you need especially if you are a post bariatric patient.

This time around, not only am I a good 127lbs, but I am healthier because I have control this time, not Dr. Jerry. He gave me the start but I am continuing this journey on my own. So if I stop and start, it's solely on me. I can restart if I stop because I know how to do so. I am on a real street called straight and I definitely have God with me. Not that I didn't before, but this time....**this time** I am wiser, smarter, stronger and tougher. I know what to expect....AND SO DO YOU!!! Make a right turn and head for the street called straight! ***

THE SKINNY GIRL STRUT

My girlfriend and I go to the movies a lot and we discuss what we are going to wear just to go to the movies. We dress up for each other. That might seem silly but it's important for a girly-girl to be a girly-girl!

Now that I am a size 6/8 we can stroll into any teen store, pull stuff off the racks and run into the dressing room together and try things on. We are in our 50's and we are acting like giggling girls. This is something that I have never, ever done. It's as if I have gotten those young teenie bopper years back. I'm playing make-up and I'm wearing over the knee boots and skinny jeans and biker-jackets and hounds-tooth suits and stripes and skinny belts and leopard cami's and I am loving getting dressed up.

You might say that you love to dress up being a large woman but there is a difference dressing up being larger and then being smaller. When you are large you have to tug and pull and sweat and snap and shove into the outfit. When you are smaller, you just put it on!

When you are skilled with make-up and you are heavy you sweat a lot and are constantly aware of getting make-up on your clothing. You are not as concerned about it when you are smaller. Now remember I am going off my own experience and those I have interviewed and witnessed from afar over a few years. You may have a different experience and that's fine.

I get dressed up for date night and I get excited to go out with my husband because I know the skinny jeans and boots are turning him on. As we walk to our seat in the movie theater, he pinches me on the butt! Wow!!!! Not that he didn't do it before, but it's a different kind of pinch, a different kind of look, a sort of, "I'm happy that you're happy," grin on his face. He even will pick me up and swing me around just as he use to do when we were teenagers in high school.

My girlfriend and I were dressed up at a Black Tie affair and we were the only ones in the Ladies Room. While we were looking in the full length mirror, we were commenting to each other how simply gorgeous we looked and as she commented on my outfit, I strutted across in front of the mirror. She said, "Girl, do your skinny girl strut!" That is where I am today, doing my skinny girl strut for the rest of my life! That's not to say that I won't begin to gain again, because life happens whether you want it to or not; but I know how to attack it and get back my strut!

I want to encourage you to go for your own strut. It will happen if you keep going.

If you happen to be a guy and have read this book for the nuggets you can get out of it, I applaud you for sticking it out to the end. You will find your "Man-Swag" as well. ***

CONCLUSION

I hope I have given you enough information to decide what you are going to do. Even though I have chosen weight lose surgery, you may not have decided to go that route but I thank you for reading this book so that you would have the information on the facts.

Weight loss is big business and we have spent billions on products that have not worked. Do what is best for you once and for all. Whether it be enrolling in a traditional program, weight loss surgery or correcting your diet and exercise, I want you to get your health in check. Now does that mean I eat EVERYTHING that's right? Nope! Right at this moment, I have my favorite candy in my purse...Sweet tarts! I may eat Oatmeal for breakfast and because I love it, I may eat it again for dinner! Oh well...that's how it goes. My husband and I might get take-out Chinese or even a bucket of Chicken when all the kids come home to visit on Sunday. But are these things every day? Absolutely not. And I know that I'll have to counter-act the junk food with healthier choices over the next few days along with exercise and more fruits, veggies and lots of water to flush it all out.

I know what I need to do to get back on that street called straight and so do you.

I would like to pray for you:

Lord, I thank you for my friend. They have decided today to do what is necessary to be in better health. Help them to walk out their desires. Help them to forgive all of the people who have ever hurt them in their life. Help them to forgive themselves for not following through on so may plans to get their health under control and to know that today is a brand new day. Help them to do what is necessary today to begin taking control of their health. Help them to look to you to be their support and to strengthen them where they are weak. Help them to know that you love them just the way that they are but that you want them to have the best health possible so that they can live the full and abundant life that you have planned for them to live.

Lord, I pray that they have an encounter with you and come to know you in a way that they have never known you before. Show them new things that will inspire them to keep going. I pray that if they don't know your Son, Jesus, they will get to know Him as their Savior and healer of the mind, the body and of the soul. And for all of their shame, Lord, give them double honor. Thank you for giving me time with them.   Amen.

You can do this! Share this book with someone you care about. May God Bless You in Your Journey,

Dr. Terri

NOTES